MODERN MEDICAL MONOGRAPHS 18

Editor in Chief: IRVING S. WRIGHT, M.D.
Consulting Editor: RICHARD H. ORR, M.D.

The Megaloblastic Anemias

By VICTOR HERBERT, M.D.

Research Assistant in Hematology,
The Mount Sinai Hospital, New
York; Presently Research Asso-
ciate, Thorndike Memorial Labo-
ratory, Boston City Hospital, and
Instructor in Medicine, Harvard
Medical School

GRUNE & STRATTON • 1959
NEW YORK AND LONDON

V

120102

The manuscript of this volume was awarded

HONORABLE MENTION

in the first Modern Medical Monographs Competition

Contents

iii

Preface

APPROXIMATELY EIGHTY YEARS AGO, Ehrlich [1] described a pathologic type of erythrocyte maturation in pernicious anemia. This
abnormal developmental line of erythrocytes was designated as
the "megaloblastic," or large germ cell, series to differentiate it
from the "normoblastic," or normal sized germ cell, series.
Anemia associated with this abnormal morphologic picture has
become known as "megaloblastic anemia."

In the eight decades since Ehrlich's first description, much has
been learned about the nature and significance of megaloblastic
blood cell formation.[2] The overwhelming majority of megaloblastic anemias have been found to be due to a deficiency of
either vitamin B_{12} or folic acid, or both vitamins.[3, 4] When a
megaloblastic morphologic picture has been observed in conditions other than frank deficiency of these vitamins, the condition
has been characterized by inhibition or exhaustion of the bone
marrow, with possible local deprivation of vitamin B_{12}, folic
acid, or building blocks for nucleoprotein synthesis in which
vitamin B_{12} and folic acid serve as co-factors. The accumulated
information has made possible a unified concept of the megaloblastic anemias as a single morphologic entity due to defective
nucleoprotein synthesis of various causes. This monograph will
be concerned with the development of megaloblastic anemia in
morphologic and biochemical terms; the causes of megaloblastic
anemia as it occurs clinically; application of this knowledge to
accurate differential diagnosis of these anemias; and a simple
and rational approach to therapy based on the actual clinical
problem, as determined by proper differential diagnosis.

This monograph is based in large measure on recent massive
and productive research in the field of the megaloblastic anemias,
carried out and reported from all parts of the globe. This is
supplemented by the author's own research experiences and observations of more than 200 cases of megaloblastic anemia seen

at the Albert Einstein College of Medicine–Bronx Municipal
Hospital Center, the Montefiore Hospital, and the Mount Sinai
Hospital, all in New York.

The author is indebted to his mentors at each of these three
eminent institutions: Dr. Irving M. London, Dr. Theodore H.
Spaet, and Dr. Louis R. Wasserman. The freedom of inquiry
and wise counsel they gave did much to make this monograph
possible. The author is also indebted to Dr. William B. Castle,
whose continued interest in the investigative work pursued by
the author was a great sustaining force.

Gratitude is also due the New York Heart Association and
Heart Fund, Inc., and its Medical Director (now retired), Dr.
D. F. Milam, for personal interest in and support of this work
from its inception, through four years of Research and Senior
Research Fellowships given to the author. Finally, and by no
means least, United States Public Health Service Research
Grants to Drs. London, Spaet, Wasserman, and the author, as
well as a grant from the National Vitamin Foundation and
various other grants, provided the equipment and supplies for
much of the research related to the megaloblastic anemias with
which the author was connected.

The author would like to thank the staff of Grune and Stratton for their patience and editorial help.

Victor Herbert, M.D.

1   *Incidence*

MEGALOBLASTIC ANEMIA is common all over the world, although the percentage of such anemias due to any specific cause varies widely from one geographic area to another and from one set of circumstances to another in any single area. As examples may be cited the prevalence of nutritional megaloblastic anemia in India,[5-8] Macedonia,[9] and Malaya [10]; the frequency of fish tapeworm megaloblastic anemia in Finland, especially widespread during World War II when particularly harsh conditions prevailed among the Finnish soldiers [11]; and the proneness of persons from the Scandinavian countries, England, Ireland, and Canada to develop classic addisonian pernicious anemia.[12]

The most common causes of megaloblastic anemia in the New York metropolitan area, where the author acquired most of his experience with the disorder, are addisonian pernicious anemia and malabsorption syndrome. The former is most common in the majority of patients; the latter predominates among the inhabitants of the city born in Puerto Rico. In all of the three New York hospitals with which the author has had major affiliation, approximately 10 per cent of the entire hematology department case load consisted of patients with megaloblastic anemia.* It is of interest in this connection that approximately the same percentage of the text of Wintrobe's *Clinical Hematology* [13] is devoted to the subject of the megaloblastic anemias, attesting to the importance of the subject to physicians in general and hematologists in particular.

The hematologic caseload of patients with megaloblastic anemia of the classic addisonian pernicious anemia variety shows every indication of a gradual future increase. This is a result of the fact that addisonian pernicious anemia is primarily a

---

* Of course, if the many cases of simple chronic anemia (as defined by Wintrobe [13]) and iron deficiency anemia which are never referred to hematology departments were so referred, the percentage of hematology department patients with megaloblastic anemia might be less than 10 per cent of the total caseload.

disease of late adult life,[14] and the average life expectancy of the population is increasing. Addisonian pernicious anemia is very rare in children,[15] rare in adults under 30 years, and seldom seen prior to the age of 40.[14]

It is presently believed that the decrease in serum vitamin B_{12} levels with aging is of dubious significance.[16] However, the increase in gastric atrophy with aging is not in doubt. Gastric atrophy may be a factor in the decrease in serum vitamin B_{12} levels and in the eventual development in some cases of megaloblastic anemia due to vitamin B_{12} deficiency.[17, 18] (See section, "Hereditarily Determined Degenerative Gastric Atrophy," page 24.)

2 *Hematologic Morphology*

IN A WELL DEVELOPED CASE of megaloblastic anemia, the picture presented by both the peripheral blood and the bone marrow is usually so characteristic as to be impossible to confuse with the morphologic picture of any other disorder. In the peripheral blood are found many large and frequently oval erythrocytes (macrocytes and macroovalocytes, the latter often referred to as "megalocytes" by European clinicians and morphologists). The nuclei of the neutrophilic polymorphonuclear leukocytes are hypersegmented,[19-21] as often are the nuclei of the eosinophils; oval neutrophils may be seen [22]; and in addition to frequently being obviously reduced in number, many of the platelets may be giant and bizarre in appearance.[23]

This picture is accompanied by a decrease in the total number of erythrocytes and neutrophilic polymorphonuclear leukocytes, and an increase in the mean corpuscular volume (MCV) of the erythrocytes due to the increased size of the average red blood cell. FIGURE 1 shows the typical appearance of the peripheral blood of a patient with megaloblastic anemia. With respect to the red blood cell morphology, it should be noted that, aside from the characteristic macrocytosis and macroovalocytosis, marked anisocytosis and poikilocytosis are frequently not present when the anemia is not severe.

The reticulocytes in the peripheral blood usually represent about 1 per cent of the total number of circulating erythrocytes. This is probably a consequence of the fact that the asynchronism in development of nucleus and cytoplasm of the erythrocyte precursors in the bone marrow results in frequent disappearance of cytoplasmic reticulum even before the nucleus is extruded. Thus more than half of the erythrocytes delivered to the peripheral blood from the bone marrow may be without reticulum. In megaloblastic anemia, therefore, the reticulocyte count provides an erroneously low figure of the rate of red cell production.[24]

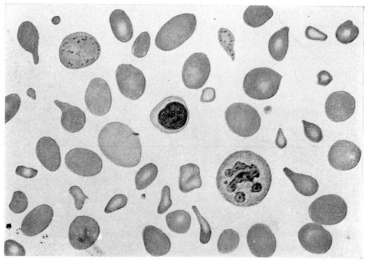

FIG. 1.—The peripheral blood in megaloblastic anemia. (From DALAND, G. A., HAM, T. H., AND PIOTTI, E.: A Color Atlas of Morphologic Hematology. Cambridge, Harvard University Press, 1951).

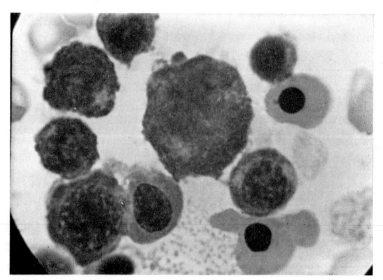

Fig. 2.—Megaloblastic development of the erythrocytes.

The bone marrow displays megaloblastic development of the erythrocytes, as shown in FIGURE 2. By comparison with normal (normoblastic) erythrocyte maturation, the megaloblastic series presents a larger size at every stage during development, with a larger amount of cytoplasm in proportion to the size of the nucleus. The nucleus itself is very large compared to the nucleus of a normoblast, and there is a striking disparity between the apparent "maturity" of the nucleus and that of the cytoplasm.[25] This disparity, or nuclear-cytoplasmic dissociation, or asynchronism, as it is variously termed,[25–27] is reflected in the much more particulate nuclear chromatin ("young nucleus," or nucleus with retarded maturation) [25, 28] of the megaloblasts at all stages of their development, even when hemoglobin is clearly visible in the cytoplasm ("old cytoplasm").[2, 29] The megaloblasts with their finely particulate "young" chromatin are easily distinguished from normoblasts with their coarsely clumped "old" nuclear chromatin, especially in those cells where hemoglobinization of the cytoplasm is visibly beginning.

Another striking feature of the bone marrow morphology in megaloblastic anemia is a megaloblastic polymorphonuclear leukopoiesis, manifested most dramatically by the presence of many giant metamyelocytes, as depicted in FIGURE 3.

There is usually a marked increase in the number of mitotic and binucleate cells in the erythroid series.

The degree of overt megaloblastosis of the bone marrow appears generally to be proportional to the severity of the anemia. Study of patients after total gastrectomy [30] demonstrated the evolutionary sequence in the development of megaloblastic anemia to be macrocytosis first, anemia second (after an average delay of one or two years following the appearance of macrocytosis), and megaloblastic marrow third and last.

Note that the first hematologic evidence of vitamin B_{12} deficiency is macrocytosis (and an Arneth count "shift to the right") with the bone marrow presumably remaining normoblastic until two or three years later. Of course, the macrocytes must have come from abnormal precursors, and in every case of early vitamin B_{12} deficiency disease which the author has seen, careful search of the bone marrow smear has revealed the presence of intermediate megaloblasts and large metamyelocytes. It is probable that these marrow findings are always present when the peripheral blood contains macroovalocytes and neutrophilic

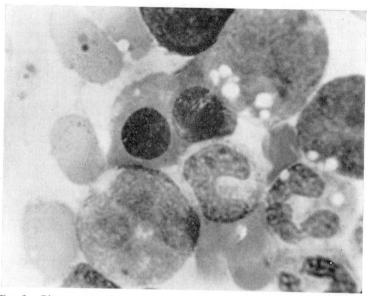

Fig. 3.—Giant metamyelocyte in a megaloblastic bone marrow. (Note also the "pinching" of the nuclei of the smaller and more mature metamyelocytes into multiple segments, resulting in the typical hypersegmented polymorphonuclear leukocytes associated with megaloblastic anemia.)

polymorphonuclear leukocytes whose nuclei show an increased amount of segmentation, even though most workers do not comment in print about abnormalities in the bone marrow until it is frankly megaloblastic. More will be said about the intermediate megaloblast shortly. For the present, suffice it to say that emphasis on the macroovalocyte and the hypersegmented polymorphonuclear leukocyte as the first indicators of a developing megaloblastic anemia is quite proper, since they are usually easily recognized and are found in the peripheral blood. Recognition of intermediate megaloblasts and large metamyelocytes, however, requires aspiration of the bone marrow and a fair amount of experience in looking at bone marrow morphology. It is wise for the person who does not examine blood and bone marrow preparations daily to compare both the peripheral blood and the bone marrow of the patient with that of a normal control subject. If he does not do this, he will miss many cases of early megaloblastic anemia, since he will not recognize the early hematologic changes.[13]

Darby et al.[31] believe that macrocytosis is the most sensitive indicator of vitamin B_{12} deficiency. Their long term observations of patients with pernicious anemia receiving smaller than minimal maintenance dosages of vitamin B_{12} indicated that the quantity of the vitamin needed for hematopoiesis exceeded that needed for other clinically recognizable physiologic functions. In the author's experience, an Arneth count "shift to the right" invariably accompanies the macrocytosis, and may even precede it.

A single case was reported suggesting that vitamin B_{12} deficiency may be manifested by an increase in the number of giant nuclei in the oral epithelial cells even before macrocytic erythrocytes make their appearance.[32] The patient had overt neurologic damage, a serum vitamin B_{12} level of 60 $\mu\mu$g./ml. (L. leishmanii assay), a serum iron concentration of 140 μg./100 ml., and definitely was not receiving folic acid therapy. It was stated that there was "no hypersegmentation of granulocytes," but an Arneth count was not reported. A photograph of the patient's peripheral blood smear was presented, and interpreted by the authors as normal except for slight anisocytosis, but it appeared suggestive of macrocytosis and at least one of the erythrocytes looked like a macroovalocyte (megalocyte). The hematocrit and red cell count were not obtained, so the MCV could not be calculated.

In the absence of folic acid administration, the author has never seen a patient having a serum vitamin B_{12} level below 100 $\mu\mu$g./ml. without incipient or overt iron deficiency who did not have at least macroovalocytosis and an Arneth count shift to the right in the peripheral blood, and at least intermediate megaloblasts and large metamyelocytes in the bone marrow.

Dr. Boen generously made the patient's original peripheral blood and bone marrow smears available for examination. The peripheral blood showed only one or two macroovalocytes per oil immersion field, but an Arneth count revealed a definite shift to the right, with 14 per cent of the neutrophilic polymorphonuclear leukocytes having more than 5 lobes. The bone marrow contained a large number of large metamyelocytes and an occasional intermediate megaloblast, but no megaloblasts. A generalized pallor of the erythrocytes suggested a possible concomitant iron deficiency despite the normal serum iron level. (Such a deficiency would explain the lack of a striking macroovalocytosis in the peripheral blood.)

Thus, this patient did have hematologic changes as well as epithelial cell changes, and the case illustrated once again the importance of the Arneth count in helping to ascertain the existence of vitamin B_{12} and/or folic acid deficiency. The question as to whether macrocytic changes due to deficiency of vitamin B_{12} may appear first in the oral epithelial cells or the hematic cells remains open. Theoretically, one would expect macrocytic changes to appear first in those cells which normally proliferate most rapidly. Concomitant iron deficiency might mask the macrocytic changes in the erythrocytes without masking the changes in the oral epithelial cells, whose iron requirement is much lower.

Recognition of the earliest hematologic signs of incipient megaloblastic anemia is particularly important because severe nervous system damage may occur in vitamin B_{12}-deficient patients prior to development of a megaloblastic marrow, and even before anemia appears.[33] The earlier such cases are recognized and proper treatment instituted, the less irreversible damage will be done. (See CHAPTER 6, "Clinical Picture," page 66, for cases in point.)

The process of development of megaloblastic anemia may take years, probably because the body is able to draw on its liver stores of vitamin B_{12} [34-38] and folinic acid [34, 39] when the exogenous supply is cut off. A simple screening procedure generally applicable to all patients on a routine basis and making it possible to recognize incipient megaloblastic anemia would be of great value. Such a procedure has long been at hand, and has been applied with marked success at the Montefiore Hospital, where in the course of a single year it increased the number of newly discovered cases of vitamin B_{12} deficiency disease from one every six weeks to one every six days.[40] In fully one-third of these cases, no anemia was present and the diagnosis was not even remotely suspected prior to the routine screening; the patients had been admitted for evaluation of unrelated conditions. The positive result of the screening procedure led to confirmation of the diagnosis of early vitamin B_{12} deficiency by determination of the serum vitamin B_{12} level and Schilling type urinary excretion testing.

This screening procedure consists simply in obtaining a routine peripheral blood smear on every new patient and carefully examining that smear for macroovalocytes and hypersegmented polymorphonuclear leukocytes. All of the technicians in the routine clinical hematology laboratory are instructed that the normal average number of lobes of the nuclei of neutrophilic polymorphonuclear leukocytes is 3; that about 40 to 50 per cent normally have 3 lobes, 20 to 40 per cent have 2 lobes, and 15 to 25 per cent have 4 lobes.[41] The finding of more than 3 5-lobed polymorphonuclears per hundred, or even a single polymorphonuclear with more than 5 lobes, or a substantial increase in the percentage with 4 lobes, signals a careful work-up for incipient megaloblastic anemia, even when absolutely no anemia is demonstrable. An increase in the number of polymorphonuclear leukocytes with 4 or more lobes, or Arneth count shift to the right,[20, 21] has preceded the onset of anemia in every case of incipient megaloblastic anemia this author has observed. Others [13] also have observed and reported on this phenomenon.

Frequently in incipient megaloblastic anemia many of the hypersegmented polymorphonuclears look at first glance like normal young polymorphonuclears with horseshoe- or sausage-shaped nuclei. More careful inspection reveals that what appears to be a single segment is in fact a rosette of overlapping segments, or rather a sausage which is being pinched into a number of small round sausages. These abnormal young polymorpho-nuclears, when in the bone marrow, are the immediate precursors of the typical hypersegmented polymorphonuclear leukocytes usually seen in the peripheral blood.[42] (See FIGURE 3.)

When macroovalocytes and hypersegmented polymorpho-nuclear leukocytes are found in the peripheral blood, examination of the bone marrow obtained by aspiration biopsy should be the next step. Even if a megaloblastic marrow is not found in such circumstances, however, work-up of the patient for an incipient megaloblastic anemia will be fruitful in the large majority of cases. It cannot be emphasized too strongly that in cases of incipient megaloblastic anemia, even highly trained hematologists may not find clearly megaloblastic primitive cells in the bone marrow. This happens despite the presence in the peripheral blood of polymorphonuclear leukocytes with hyper-segmented nuclei and occasional macroovalocytes, which testify to the fact that some megaloblastic hematopoiesis must be taking place, and despite subsequent confirmation of this diagnosis by determination of the serum vitamin B_{12} level [17] (which may often be in the "low normal" range), and the Schilling test. (See CHAPTER 6, "Clinical Picture," page 10, for cases in point.)

A recent report [43] calls attention to the possible usefulness of discriminating from megaloblasts "lines of red cell development morphologically intermediate between unequivocal megalo-blastic erythropoiesis and normoblastic erythropoiesis" (i.e., "intermediate megaloblasts").[26, 44, 45] The authors of that report believe that this modified type of megaloblastic erythropoiesis represents the morphologic result of the combination of a condition that would usually produce a megaloblastic marrow and an associated iron deficiency at the marrow level.

Actually, as eminent authorities [46, 47, 38A] have noted, "inter-mediate megaloblasts," or "macroblasts," [17] may be simply erythrocyte precursors with a supply of vitamin B_{12} or folic acid which is insufficient for normal maturation but not so grossly inadequate as to result in complete megaloblastosis. They are characteristic of minor or partial deficiencies of vitamin B_{12} or folic acid. Intermediate megaloblasts, along with large but not quite giant metamyelocytes, are often the only observable abnormality in the bone marrow of patients who are not yet severely anemic, but who do have overt macroovalocytosis and an increase in the number of hypersegmented polymorphonuclear leukocytes in the peripheral blood. The author has seen intermediate megaloblastic erythropoiesis in a number of cases of pure vitamin B_{12} or folic acid deficiency, during the period of slight anemia which precedes the full blown clinical picture of megaloblastic anemia, as well as early in the period of response to therapy. No associated iron deficiency existed in these cases.

In all 4 cases of the report mentioned,[43] hypersegmented polymorphonuclear leukocytes and macrocytes were noted in the peripheral blood, indicating the existence of an underlying megaloblastic erythropoiesis which was manifested in the bone marrow by intermediate megaloblastic erythrocyte development. It is true that associated iron deficiency often results in an intermediate megaloblastic bone marrow morphology. This is the product of interaction of the tendency toward megaloblastosis induced by folic acid or vitamin B_{12} deficiency and the tendency toward microcytosis induced by iron deficiency. These cases,[43] along with others in which evaluation of the bone marrow morphology may be difficult, further confirm the significance of the presence in the peripheral blood of both macrocytes and hypersegmented polymorphonuclear leukocytes in increased numbers.

The intermediate megaloblasts observed in combined iron and vitamin B_{12} (or folic acid) deficiency are readily converted to overt megaloblasts by iron therapy. Conversely, vitamin B_{12} (or folic acid) therapy will convert the normochromic cells to hypochromic cells.

The presence in the peripheral blood of either macrocytes or an increased number of hypersegmented polymorphonuclear leukocytes alone is of less significance in diagnosing possible megaloblastic anemia, actual or incipient, than the presence of both together. Reticulocytes are large red cells, and an increased number of reticulocytes may convey an erroneous impression that macrocytosis is present. A variable number of macrocytes (and infrequently even some macroovalocytes) are part of the anisocytosis and poikilocytosis which accompany many diseases, especially those of a primarily hematologic nature. Macrocytosis is a frequent accompaniment of liver disease [13, 13a] and aplastic anemia; these subjects will be discussed subsequently.

An increased number of polymorphonuclear leukocytes with hypersegmented nuclei is less commonly seen than are macrocytes in conditions other than those leading to a megaloblastic anemia, but they do appear with sepsis and widespread malignancy (especially the leukemias), and characterize the interesting familial entity of "constitutional hypersegmentation of the neutrophil nucleus." [48] When both macroovalocytes and hypersegmented polymorphonuclears in increased numbers are clearly present, an incipient or actual megaloblastic anemia is the most likely cause.

It may well be that the hypersegmented polymorphonuclear leukocytes very occasionally seen with sepsis and widespread malignancy are in fact products of folic acid deficiency at the bone marrow level caused by extremely rapid cell turnover.

The hematologic features of vitamin B_{12} or folic acid deficiency are frequently partly masked by coincident iron deficiency.[3, 48a] Most frequently, this masking takes the form of a *dimorphic* peripheral blood picture, with some red cells macrocytic and usually fully hemoglobinated but sometimes hypochromic, and others microcytic and hypochromic.[49, 384] Sometimes the microcytes of iron deficiency appear to "cancel out" the macrocytes of vitamin B_{12} or folic acid deficiency, and the patient's peripheral blood picture is that of a normocytic normochromic or hypochromic anemia. If the iron deficiency is of sufficient severity, one may observe in the peripheral blood only a hypochromic microcytic anemia, with no macroovalocytes present.[13]

In the author's experience, despite the severity of the iron deficiency, and despite partial or complete obliteration of macro-ovalocytes in the peripheral blood in the presence of vitamin B_{12} or folic acid deficiency, *the increase in number of neutro-philic polymorphonuclear leukocytes with hypersegmented nuclei is not masked,* and provides a clue to the coexistence of vitamin B_{12} or folic acid deficiency with the iron deficiency. (See FIGURE 4.)

The author has seen such patients (often pregnant or with a malabsorption syndrome) with concomitant iron deficiency and vitamin B_{12} deficiency, often with associated folic acid

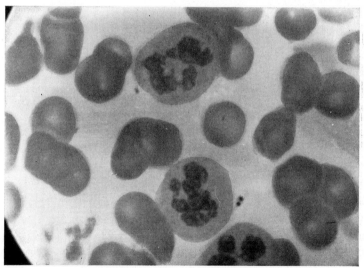

FIG. 4.—Typical hypersegmented polymorphonuclear leukocytes due to vitamin B_{12} deficiency in the peripheral blood of a patient who did not have macro-ovalocytosis (or even macrocytosis) because of the concomitant iron deficiency. In this case, a normocytic normochromic anemia was present, due to a perfect "cancelling out" by each deficiency of the erythrocyte morphology caused by the other deficiency. Serum vitamin $B_{12} = 90$ $\mu\mu$g./ml.; serum iron $= 110$ μg. per cent. Hematocrit $= 28$ per cent; hemoglobin $= 9.4$ Gm./100 ml.; red cell count $= 3.2$ million/cu.mm.; MCV $= 87.5$ μ^3; MCHC $= 34\%$. After vitamin B_{12} treatment, serum iron fell to 26 μg. per cent and hypochromic microcytic anemia appeared.

deficiency, in whose peripheral blood striking hypochromia was present along with an increase in the number of polymorphonuclear leukocytes with hypersegmented nuclei, but with no macroovalocytosis. Presented with such a case, outstanding hematologists have ignored the hypersegmented polymorphonuclears (and the intermediate megaloblasts and large metamyelocytes in the bone marrow), and have made a diagnosis of uncomplicated iron deficiency anemia. These diagnoses were subsequently proved wrong by determination of the serum vitamin B_{12} level to be below 100 $\mu\mu g./ml.$, the serum "folic acid" level to be below 5 $m\mu g./ml.$, and development of overt megaloblastic anemia with macroovalocytosis after iron therapy, and cure by administration of vitamin B_{12} (and folic acid when required). Deficiency of both iron and vitamin B_{12} without concomitant folic acid deficiency may be noted after total gastrectomy (and occasionally after distal subtotal gastrectomy), with terminal ileitis or other secondary malabsorption states, in elderly patients with histamine-refractory achlorhydria and anemia,[48a] and as a result of two separate disorders coincidentally occurring in the same patient. An example of the latter is the coincidental occurrence of pernicious anemia and gastrointestinal tract bleeding.

Thus, in the presence of hypochromic erythrocytes in the peripheral blood, it is wise to suspect a concomitant megaloblastic anemia, even if no macroovalocytes are present, when one observes an increased number of hypersegmented polymorphonuclear leukocytes, especially when intermediate megaloblasts and large metamyelocytes are present in the bone marrow. It is possible that in conditions other than iron deficiency, but also characterized by defective hemoglobin synthesis, macroovalocytes may also be absent despite the presence of a coincidental vitamin B_{12} or folic acid deficiency.

Even when the erythrocytes appear normochromic, it is wise to suspect vitamin B_{12} or folic acid deficiency with associated iron deficiency if there is an increased number of polymorphonuclear leukocytes with nuclei containing more than three lobes.

3   *The Biochemical Basis of Megaloblastic Hematopoiesis*

BIOCHEMICAL STUDIES OF MEGALOBLASTS have been directed in two main channels: (1) quantitative chemical studies to determine the differences in content between megaloblasts and normoblasts; and (2) studies of the biochemical mechanisms whereby the differences in content occur.

It has been determined that the large amount of cytoplasm of the megaloblast contains considerably more ribonucleic acid (RNA) than the cytoplasm of the normoblast [50, 51]; this is true at all stages of maturation, and is most striking when hemoglobinization is occurring and RNA is almost gone from the normoblast but still persists in significant concentration in the megaloblast.

The large nucleus of the megaloblast has been estimated to contain as much as double the amount of deoxyribonucleic acid (DNA) as the normoblast nucleus,[52] though not all workers agree that the DNA level of the megaloblast is so high.[29] There is a fairly definite increase in the RNA:DNA ratio of the megaloblast [52]; this is reflected in an increased uracil:thymine ratio.[53]

Feulgen-stained smears of megaloblasts demonstrated their nuclear chromatin to be present in smaller particles than that of normoblasts.[29]

With the demonstration that in the mammal uridine may be incorporated into thymidine,[54] it was possible to conceive of cytoplasmic RNA as the principal source of material for nuclear DNA, and further to suggest that any failure of utilization of RNA to provide material for DNA formation would lead to a persistence of cytoplasmic RNA resulting in macrocyte production.[2] In this schema, any retardation of DNA synthesis to the twice-resting-cell concentration required for mitosis would cause the marrow to become crowded with cells waiting to divide, and slowly building up their DNA content while a large backlog of RNA builds up in the cytoplasm. Biochemical evidence of blockage in pyrimidine nucleotide formation in vitamin B_{12} deficiency continues to be gathered.[54a]

The megaloblast may thus be explained as a young red blood cell resulting from a prolonged phase between mitoses * allowing a longer time for dispersion of the chromatin throughout the nucleus,[2, 25, 55] thus producing its typical finely particulate appearance. Anything which retards the rate of cell division could therefore cause megaloblasts to be produced.

The concept of the megaloblast as a product of "retardation of the nuclear evolution by blockage of the mitoses of maturation" has been repeatedly stressed in the literature, and recently thoroughly reviewed by Cazal,[25] and by Reisner.[2] It would seem that any retardation of cellular proliferation would be manifested not only in the hematopoietic system, but also in other areas where the production of new cells is normally rapid. Such indeed is the case, as demonstrated by the presence of "megaloblastic" oral, gastric, and vaginal epithelial cells in patients with pernicious anemia.[32, 56-58]

Similar alterations in gastric cytology have been described in pernicious anemia and in sprue.[59] Such similarities may be interpreted as the *effect* of inadequate absorption of vitamin B_{12} (and folic acid), and other deficiencies. Interpreting them as a *cause* of the inadequate absorption would be hazardous.

In practical clinical terms, megaloblastic blood formation is observed nearly always in the presence of inadequate amounts of vitamin B_{12}, folic acid, or both. After the isolation of folic acid in 1943,[61, 62] and vitamin B_{12} in 1948,[63, 64] it was possible to study the role of these two agents in nucleoprotein synthesis.

Both of these agents function in the metabolism of one-carbon units: folic acid primarily as a carrier of hydroxymethyl and formyl groups [65] and in formimino group transfer [66]; vitamin B_{12} in the *de novo* synthesis of labile methyl groups.[67] These vitamins are therefore essential in the synthesis of purines and pyrimidines,[68-70, 70a] which are integral parts of RNA and DNA

---

* It should be noted that arrest of mitosis of cultured chick embryo osteoblasts and fibroblasts induced by folic acid antagonists occurs in metaphase.[60]

molecules. Vitamin B_{12} influences folic acid metabolism,[71] but there is no evidence at present that folic acid directly influences vitamin B_{12} metabolism.

When a patient with a megaloblastic anemia is treated with vitamin B_{12} or folic acid, depending on his primary deficiency, the RNA:DNA ratio rapidly falls to normal.[72] In pernicious anemia bone marrow cultures, vitamin B_{12} speeds up the production of DNA.[73] The speed of these phenomena explains the rapidity with which the megaloblastic marrow converts to normoblastic on institution of treatment; almost complete conversion usually occurs within 24 to 48 hours. If conversion does not occur with the anticipated speed, either complications are present or the wrong agent is being used. (Temporary responses may be obtained with folic acid in vitamin B_{12} deficiency states, or conversely vitamin B_{12} in folic acid deficiency states, but eventually the patient becomes refractory to the wrong agent, presumably as a result of complete exhaustion of his remaining stores of the vitamin in which he was deficient.)

Biochemical studies have done much in the way of delineating the mechanism of megaloblastic blood formation, but many questions still remain unanswered. It is presently accepted that folic acid deficiency leads directly to megaloblastic anemia; it is not yet certain that vitamin B_{12} deficiency is a direct cause of the disease. The question is still open as to whether the megaloblastic anemia which follows vitamin B_{12} deprivation is a direct result solely of such deprivation or is partly the result of deranged folic acid metabolism caused by deficiency of vitamin B_{12}.

In this connection, it is of interest that 5 to 10 mg. of folic acid daily (10 to 20 times the rough minimal daily maintenance requirement) will usually produce hematologic remission in previously untreated patients with vitamin B_{12} deficiency, whereas as much as 1000 μg. of vitamin B_{12} daily (perhaps 1000 times the rough minimal daily maintenance requirement) is often inadequate to produce hematologic remission in patients with primary folic acid deficiency.

4 *Etiologic Classification of the Megaloblastic Anemias Due to Vitamin B₁₂ Deficiency*

As STATED IN THE PREFACE, the presence of a megaloblastic anemia is almost pathognomonic of a deficiency of vitamin B_{12}, folic acid, or both. Failure adequately to ingest, absorb, utilize, or retain either or both of these vitamins accounts for nearly every case of megaloblastic anemia. The small percentage of cases which have not yet been demonstrated to be a result of a deficiency in availability of either of these vitamins at the bone marrow level is almost uniformly characterized by inhibition or exhaustion of the bone marrow. It may well be that the megaloblastosis in these conditions will prove to be caused by interference with utilization or local exhaustion of the supply of vitamin B_{12} or folic acid at the bone marrow level.

Since deficiency of vitamin B_{12} or of folic acid directly or indirectly underlies nearly all, if not all, of the clearly megaloblastic anemias recorded in the literature at the present time, classification of these anemias in terms of etiology of the deficiency simplifies understanding, allows a methodological approach to differential diagnosis, and insures appropriate therapy.

I. INADEQUATE INGESTION

The daily dietary requirement of the adult for vitamin B_{12} is approximately 1 μg. This assumption is based on the facts that a daily parenteral dose of 1 μg. induces remission in pernicious anemia,[74, 75] and a similar amount of the vitamin provides a minimal maintenance dosage.[31, 71, 76]

Vitamin B_{12} is synthesized by microorganisms, and is found in the tissue and fluid stores of marine and animal life which ingests such microorganisms. Therefore, the sources of vitamin B_{12} in the human diet are the protein-rich animal products. Liver and kidney, and sea food such as oysters and clams, are especially rich in this vitamin. Other dietary sources include all meats and sea food, and to a lesser degree eggs, milk, and milk products.[77-79] Failure to ingest an adequate quantity of animal protein will eventually lead to vitamin B$_{12}$ deficiency.

A. Vegans

Vegans are strict ovolacto-vegetarians who subsist on a diet devoid of animal protein, including dairy products and eggs. The eventual development of vitamin B$_{12}$ deficiency in such individuals has been documented by Wokes, Badenoch, and Sinclair.[80] The vegan, whose diet is adequate in folic and ascorbic acid content, provides the best instance of "pure" nutritional vitamin B$_{12}$ deficiency. The other nutritional vitamin B$_{12}$ deficiency states are associated with multiple other dietary deficiencies, often including folic and ascorbic acids, and it is difficult to determine to what extent megaloblastic anemia is caused by lack of folic and ascorbic acids in such cases (see C).

B. Chronic Alcoholism

Prolonged alcoholism with a concomitant reduction in ingestion of vitamin B$_{12}$-containing foods may result in overt vitamin B$_{12}$ deficiency.[81-83] When cirrhosis is associated with the chronic alcoholism, the development of a megaloblastic anemia is more likely a reflection of folic acid deficiency than of vitamin B$_{12}$ deficiency.[84] (See section, "Cirrhosis Associated with Chronic Alcoholism," page 52.)

C. Poverty, Religious Tenets, Ignorance, Dietary Faddism

Poverty, with ingestion of a diet containing very little animal protein, such as the bread, olives, beans, and tomatoes which made up the diet of the Macedonians studied by Fairley et al.,[9] results in vitamin B$_{12}$ deficiency, along with multiple other deficiencies. Abstention from animal protein on religious grounds will also produce vitamin B$_{12}$ deficiency if the abstention is complete.[13, 85] The author has observed pure nutritional vitamin B_{12} deficiency in a 20 year old Columbia University student from India who ate no animal protein for religious reasons. He had megaloblastic anemia, a serum vitamin B_{12} level of 49 $\mu\mu$g./ml. (E. gracilis), a normal serum "folic acid" level of 8 mμg./ml. (L. casei), and no urinary excretion of formiminoglutamic acid.

A similar phenomenon may sometimes be observed in elderly persons who live alone and eat little except for easy to prepare carbohydrate foods,[86] and in certain dietary faddists.[87]

However, all of the patients of whom the author is aware who had megaloblastic anemia associated with *grossly* inadequate diets, had folic acid deficiency, manifested usually with normal serum vitamin B_{12} levels and very low serum "folic acid" levels. (See section, "Nutritional Megaloblastic Anemia," page 51.)

D. Hyperthyroidism

Hyperthyroidism has been reported in association with megaloblastic anemia in two series of cases.[88, 89] It is possible this association may be a consequence of increased demand for and turnover of vitamin B_{12} in thyrotoxicosis,[90, 91] in the presence of a marginal dietary intake, especially since the anemia may disappear after subtotal thyroidectomy.[92] The concomitant requirement of marginal intake for vitamin B_{12} deficiency to develop would explain the low incidence of megaloblastic anemia among thyrotoxic patients.

II. DEFECTIVE ABSORPTION

The majority of cases of megaloblastic anemia due to vitamin B_{12} deficiency fall into the various categories of this classification.

There appear to be two separate and distinct mechanisms for absorption of vitamin B_{12}.[93–95] With physiologic doses of vitamin B_{12} (that is, amounts of 0.5 to 2 μg., as found in the average American meal [96]), absorption is dependent upon intrinsic factor.[97] This normal pattern of absorption is the one of utmost clinical significance, for it is interference with this pattern that produces the megaloblastic anemias resulting from failure to absorb vitamin B_{12}.

The other mechanism of absorption is independent of intrinsic factor, but is primarily operative only in the presence of supraphysiologic doses of vitamin B_{12} (that is, amounts much greater than those found in the usual diet). A significant aliquot of such doses is absorbed by a "mass action" effect, possibly diffusion.[93-95] This mechanism has clinical significance primarily in oral therapy of vitamin B_{12} deficiency, and will be discussed further in that connection.

A. Inadequate or Absent Secretion of Intrinsic Factor

The prototype of all the megaloblastic anemias is addisonian pernicious anemia, described as an etiological entity by Sir Thomas Addison in 1855,[98] and Biermer in 1872.[99] Subsequent expansion of knowledge led to the realization that the megaloblastic anemias were not an etiologic entity, but rather the similar clinical and pathologic result of various causes. At the present time the term "pernicious anemia" (or "addisonian pernicious anemia") is reserved in the Anglo-American literature for that megaloblastic anemia characterized by an idiopathic deficiency of Castle's intrinsic factor.[55] In other countries the term "pernicious anemia" is given a wider interpretation, and includes all of the "pure" vitamin B_{12} deficiency states.[100]

Following hard on the heels of Minot and Murphy's Nobel prize-winning discovery that a diet high in liver produced remission in 45 patients with pernicious anemia,[101] Castle and his associates [102-105] demonstrated that beef cattle muscle (an animal protein) contained an "extrinsic (food) factor" which interacted with an "intrinsic factor" in normal human gastric juice to yield an "anti-pernicious anemia principle" which restored hematopoiesis to normal when given orally to the pernicious anemia patient. The oral administration of either extrinsic factor or intrinsic factor alone had no effect.

Two decades later, vitamin B_{12} was demonstrated to be the extrinsic factor,[106] and also to be the anti-pernicious anemia principle.[107] Since vitamin B_{12} is the anti-pernicious anemia principle, and is fully effective in treating pernicious anemia when administered parenterally, the role of intrinsic factor appears to be that of effecting the transfer of ingested vitamin B_{12} across the intestinal mucosa and into the blood stream.[55] Whether the vitamin B_{12} is absorbed alone, or the vitamin B_{12}-intrinsic factor combination is absorbed, has not yet been determined. Favoring the latter possibility is a report of the presence in human serum of a substance similar to intrinsic factor.[108, 109] Furthermore, there is some experimental evidence that receptors for intrinsic factor may exist in both intestinal mucosa [108–115] and liver,[108–110] and that intrinsic factor may be involved in the selective deposition of vitamin B_{12} in the liver.[108–110] This work requires confirmation and extension before general acceptance.

The chemical nature of intrinsic factor is not known, since this substance has not been isolated in pure form. It is probably a mucoprotein or mucopolypeptide.[116–119] In man, the glandular structure of the fundus and cardiac portions of the stomach is the site of intrinsic factor secretion.[120, 121] In the rat, the chief (pepsinogen) cells of the fundus glands probably are the intrinsic factor elaborating cells.[122]

1. Failure of the Stomach to Adequately Secrete Intrinsic Factor

a. Addisonian Pernicious Anemia

This term includes all of the megaloblastic anemias of vitamin B_{12} deficiency resulting from inadequate secretion of intrinsic factor in which the basic cause of this deficient secretion is unknown. In these cases the gastric mucosa rarely may be histologically normal, but usually shows gastric atrophy or an atrophic gastritis of varying severity.[123–126]

Extensive study of patients with fish tapeworm vitamin B_{12}

deficiency [127] has revealed that with the vitamin B_{12} deficiency a variable degree of gastric atrophy develops, and a variable degree of reversion of the histologic picture of the stomach toward normal accompanies the therapy. This would suggest that in some instances vitamin B_{12} deficiency may be the cause, rather than the result, of gastric atrophy. Prolonged iron deficiency may also cause gastric atrophy,[128] eventuating in loss of intrinsic factor secretion and addisonian pernicious anemia.[129]

Addisonian pernicious anemia is itself probably not an etiologic entity, but rather a syndrome of several possible etiologies which will be detailed below:

(1). *Hereditarily determined failure of intrinsic factor secretion.* The physiologic mechanism responsible for stimulating gastric secretion of intrinsic factor is unknown. Inadequate functioning of this mechanism or of the equally unknown enzymatic mechanism of production of intrinsic factor is responsible for the most widely studied form of pernicious anemia, with the possible exception of that anemia resulting from degenerative gastric atrophy.

Hereditarily determined primary failure of gastric secretion of intrinsic factor has been inferred from the rare cases of pernicious anemia in childhood,[15, 130] pernicious anemia without achlorhydria,[131–133] the high association coefficient of these two types of pernicious anemia, the high familial tendency of the disease,[134–136] and its occurrence in monovular twins.[137]

Harris-Jones, Swan, and Tudhope [138] have reported the case of a 16 year old girl with megaloblastic anemia whose baseline secretion of intrinsic factor was inadequate. Parenteral administration of the powerful secretagogue and parasympathetic stimulant Carbachol (carbamylcholine chloride) induced secretion of a normal quantity of intrinsic factor. Previously, Mollin, Baker, and Doniach [123] had reported a similar case in a young man; in their case the deficient baseline secretion of intrinsic factor was only partly correctible by administration of Carbachol.

In some individuals the usual secretion of intrinsic factor under physiologic circumstances is low, though these individuals may have normal serum vitamin B_{12} levels and histologically normal gastric mucosa. Carbachol stimulation evoked normal secretion of intrinsic factor in a group of such subjects, but one of them was eventually unable to secrete intrinsic factor even after such stimulation, and was then classified as a case of pernicious anemia.[139, 140] A possibly similar such case is now under observation.[141]

Study of patients diagnosed as having pernicious anemia in the 1930's revealed that many had small amounts of intrinsic factor in their gastric juice.[142] It is not possible as yet to delineate the exact etiology of the megaloblastic anemia resulting from idiopathic (and most probably hereditary[143, 144]) failure of secretion of intrinsic factor; the evidence at present indicates it results from an enzymatic defect in the production of intrinsic factor, resulting in inadequate production and eventual total cessation of production. Primary inadequacy of the *stimulus* to intrinsic factor secretion has not yet been excluded as an etiologic factor, however.

(2). *Hereditarily determined degenerative gastric atrophy.* A genetically determined tendency to develop gastric atrophy with aging has been well documented,[143–145] as has the frequent (but not uniform) association of gastric atrophy and failure of intrinsic factor secretion.[126, 143–147] The possible relation of this entity to (1) above and (3) below is undetermined, but its frequency of occurrence is high.

(3). *Gastric atrophy as the end stage of superficial inflammatory gastritis; superficial gastritis with atrophy.* Pernicious anemia has been observed in gastric atrophy resulting from chronic gastritis,[148] and associated with superficial gastritis with atrophy, atrophic gastritis of varying severity, and gastric atrophy in which relationship to gastritis was not established.[125, 149] Whether these different types of lesions in adult pernicious anemia are stages in the same pathological process and closely related to (1) and (2) above, or distinct etiologic entities falling into separate categories of atrophic gastritis and gastric atrophy remains to be seen.[125] It has already been mentioned that prolonged iron [128] or vitamin B_{12} [127] deficiency may produce gastric atrophy; that atrophy passes through stages of gastritis before being established. Serial studies of the gastric mucosa in large numbers of living patients will be needed to clarify these relationships.

b. Lesions Which Destroy the Gastric Mucosa

Ingested corrosives,[150] linitis plastica of non-neoplastic origin,[151] and extensive neoplastic disease [152] may each destroy the intrinsic factor-secreting glandular lining of the stomach and thereby eventually produce a megaloblastic anemia due to vitamin B_{12} deficiency.

Neoplastic disease producing megaloblastic anemia must be separated from gastric carcinoma arising in patients with pernicious anemia. The incidence of gastric carcinoma in autopsied patients with both pernicious anemia and gastric atrophy is about 10 to 12 per cent; this is more than three times the expected occurrence of gastric carcinoma at autopsy.[153–155] The high coincidence of gastric carcinoma and pernicious anemia is probably a consequence of the fact that both conditions frequently arise from a common genetically determined gastric atrophy,[144, 145] or perhaps that the gastric atrophy which results in pernicious anemia is also associated with intestinal metaplasia in the body area of the stomach [125] which may be a precancerous lesion. In a given patient with carcinoma of the fundus or body of the stomach with gastric atrophy and pernicious anemia, it is impossible at present to determine *post hoc* which came first.

c. Endocrine Disorders

Pituitary and gonadal insufficiency have been reported to produce infrequently a pernicious anemia-like picture, leading to the suggestion that a hormonal inadequacy may lead to degeneration of the intrinsic factor-producing cells.[156]

In the few cases of hypothyroidism in which a megaloblastic anemia has appeared and causes of megaloblastic anemia unrelated to hypothyroidism have been excluded, it has appeared to result from defective intestinal absorption of vitamin B_{12}, unrelated to secretion of intrinsic factor.[157] However, there may be a depressed secretion of intrinsic factor in some cases.[157, 158]

Addison's disease has also on rare occasions been reported in association with pernicious anemia.[159, 160] The relation of these two conditions is obscure.

2. Gastrectomy

a. Total

Total gastrectomy removes the source of intrinsic factor [161] and will invariably eventually produce megaloblastic anemia due to vitamin B_{12} deficiency if appropriate prophylaxis with vitamin B_{12} is not instituted.[30] The period of time which will elapse before development of anemia will depend on the amount of the body stores of vitamin B_{12} and on the dietary content of vitamin B_{12} and folic acid.

b. Subtotal

(1). *Proximal.* Proximal subtotal gastrectomy with esophagoantrostomy may ablate the intrinsic factor-secreting glands to such an extent as to produce vitamin B_{12} deficiency.[162] Less extensive proximal subtotal gastrectomy is seldom followed by inadequate intrinsic factor secretion.[163]

(2). *Distal.* Distal subtotal gastrectomy is performed much more frequently than proximal subtotal gastrectomy. In a survey of over 1500 patients who had this operation performed, MacLean [162] found that only 9 patients subsequently developed a megaloblastic anemia associated with a hemoglobin below 10 Gm./100 ml. In every one of these 9 patients, histologic review of the resected portion of the stomach demonstrated a gastric atrophy. This suggested that these 9 patients would eventually have developed a megaloblastic anemia due to lack of intrinsic factor even if subtotal gastrectomy had not been performed, and that the subtotal gastrectomy had no relation to the development of the megaloblastic anemia.

Previously,[164] 5 patients had been reported with megaloblastic anemia developing from 2 to 12 years after subtotal gastrectomy, accompanied by inadequate vitamin B$_{12}$ absorption correctible by oral administration of intrinsic factor. Of these 5 patients 4 had atrophy of the gastric mucosa as demonstrated by examination of a gastric biopsy, despite the fact that such atrophy was not present at the time of gastrectomy. The authors of that report noted that the patients were originally operated upon because of gastric ulcer, which may itself have led to gastritis and eventual atrophy with loss of intrinsic factor secretion.

Loewenstein [163] noted low vitamin B$_{12}$ absorption in 3 of 22 patients who had distal subtotal gastrectomy. All 3 patients were tested for B$_{12}$ absorption ability more than 6 years after operation, whereas most of the other 19 patients were tested less than 6 years after operation. None of the 3 patients with low B$_{12}$ absorption had macrocytic anemia; in fact, 2 had hypochromic microcytic anemia associated with a low serum iron concentration, i.e., iron deficiency anemia. All 3 had gastro*jejunostomies* after their gastric resection.

Still more recently,[165] decreased absorption of vitamin B$_{12}$, correctible by oral administration of intrinsic factor, was found in 4 of 19 patients who had had subtotal gastrectomy followed by gastro*jejunostomy,* but in none of 15 patients who had had subtotal gastrectomy followed by gastro*duodenostomy.* None of the 34 subjects had anemia. The surgical specimens at gastrectomy of 3 of the 4 patients with subsequently decreased vitamin B$_{12}$ absorption had normal gastric mucosa.

Putting these various findings together, it seems that following distal subtotal gastrectomy, especially if it is followed by gastrojejunostomy rather than gastroduodenostomy, gastric secretion of intrinsic factor may be diminished.[165] In the course of a number of years, atrophy may develop in the gastric remnant, with loss of residual ability to secrete intrinsic factor.[164] Mild vitamin B$_{12}$ deficiency may occur not infrequently, but severe megaloblastic anemia, as a direct result of the distal subtotal gastrectomy uncomplicated by other factors, is rare. A complicating factor might be the occasional development of a malabsorption syndrome after partial gastrectomy.[165a] In this connection, there is a greater rapidity of gastric emptying and intestinal transit after subtotal gastrectomy. This is more marked after a Billroth II procedure (gastro*jejunostomy*) than after a Billroth I operation (gastro*duodenostomy*).[165b]

If the absorption of iron occurs chiefly in the duodenal region,[13, 166, 166a] iron deficiency should be expected to occur more frequently when subtotal gastrectomy is followed by gastrojejunostomy than when it is followed by gastroduodenostomy. Long-continued iron deficiency itself may then lead to gastric atrophy and intrinsic factor deficiency.[128, 129, 167]

When any patient undergoes subtotal gastrectomy, the extent of the gastric remnant should be clearly and precisely recorded, as should the appearance of the mucosa of the resected portion. The patient must be closely checked for the possible development of iron deficiency. His ability to absorb a test dose of radioactive vitamin B_{12} should be determined about two months after operation.[165] If poor, and correctible by oral administration of intrinsic factor, the patient should be treated for the rest of his life just as if he had pernicious anemia. If his ability to absorb vitamin B_{12} is normal, the patient should have semiannual examinations of his peripheral blood smear and determination of his hematocrit, hemoglobin, and red cell count, along with serum iron and vitamin B_{12} determinations, if available. It is probably in the patient's best interest to continue such semiannual examinations for at least 10 years after the subtotal gastrectomy. As stated previously, however, the incidence of megaloblastic anemia after subtotal gastrectomy is quite low, even in patients followed for a number of years.

3. Intrinsic Factor Inhibitor in Gastric Secretion

A recent preliminary report [168] presented "an unusual case of pernicious anemia diagnosed in a male at the age of 13 months with a 25 year follow-up." The patient consistently had free acid and very high urinary uropepsin levels. The anemia responded to intramuscular injections of vitamin B$_{12}$, but not to oral administration of the vitamin together with intrinsic factor. Radioactive vitamin B$_{12}$ studies demonstrated extremely poor intestinal absorption, not influenced by addition of intrinsic factor, normal gastric juice, or bowel sterilization with tetracycline. Since "five hundred ml. of the patient's gastric juice plus vitamin B$_{12}$ and intrinsic factor given orally to a woman with a subtotal gastrectomy and with normal B$_{12}$ absorption depressed her absorption of B$_{12}$ by 50%," the authors concluded that "this patient's gastric juice, in sufficient quantity, will inhibit the absorption of B$_{12}$ from the intestinal tract, causing a variant of pernicious anemia."

However, there is evidence that large amounts of intrinsic factor given orally, such as the 500 ml. of gastric juice plus additional intrinsic factor in the form of a hog intrinsic factor concentrate, which was given to the woman with a subtotal gastrectomy, may inhibit the absorption of vitamin B$_{12}$ in any recipient.[112, 169-173] Therefore production of inhibited absorption with such a large dose of intrinsic factor-containing material does not constitute an argument in favor of the existence of an intrinsic factor inhibitor in the gastric juice that was given. Furthermore, if such an inhibitor did exist, it might be expected that it could be overcome (although this is not necessarily true) by a large dose of intrinsic factor. The authors report, however, that "massive dosage of intrinsic factor given orally did not correct the absorptive defect."

The validity of the contention that the patient's gastric juice contains an intrinsic factor inhibitor cannot yet be considered proved. A mild form of coeliac disease or a selective malabsorption for vitamin B$_{12}$ remain major diagnostic possibilities. A search for evidences of malabsorption for other agents remains to be reported, as does the result of oral administration of a *moderate* amount (25 to 100 ml.) of the patient's gastric juice with radioactive vitamin B$_{12}$ to a recipient with known addisonian pernicious anemia, both in the absence and in the presence of added hog intrinsic factor concentrate.

Nevertheless, the speculation that some individuals may have an inhibitor of intrinsic factor in their gastric juice is interesting, and worth keeping in mind. There is some evidence that such an inhibitor may exist, in the form of degraded or incomplete intrinsic factor unable to bind vitamin B_{12} but able to attach to intestinal receptors and block their uptake of intrinsic factor.[173a]

B. Small Intestinal Disorder

Variable degrees of reduced absorption of vitamin B_{12} and of folic acid may occur with any structural or functional disorder affecting the small intestine.

The absorption of physiologic amounts of vitamin B_{12} occurs primarily in the small intestine. This has been demonstrated by instillation of radioactive vitamin B_{12} through an intestinal tube directly into the duodenum, jejunum, and ileum.[174] It is probable that no significant absorption occurs from the stomach, since oral administration of normal gastric juice with vitamin B_{12} to gastrectomized patients is not only effective, but may actually produce greater vitamin B_{12} absorption than that observed on similar treatment of patients with pernicious anemia whose stomachs are intact.[175] Bypassing the stomach by duodenal intubation [174] or timed release capsules [176] has also resulted in greater vitamin B_{12} absorption than that observed when the stomach was not bypassed. Possible explanations for this phenomenon include binding of vitamin B_{12} by materials in the stomach that have no intrinsic factor activity,[119, 173a, 177–179] and the adverse affect of acid pH on vitamin B_{12} absorption.[112, 180]

It is probable that most vitamin B_{12} absorption in man occurs in the ileum,[140, 181, 182] as it does in the rat [182–185] and the dog.[186] There is practically no absorption of vitamin B_{12} by patients who have had all their small intestine except the jejunum resected.[140, 181]

No significant absorption of vitamin B_{12} occurs from the colon, as proved by direct instillation of vitamin B$_{12}$ into the colon,[174] and the fact that the stools of patients with pernicious anemia contain large amounts of vitamin B$_{12}$ synthesized by bacteria in the colon, which would produce remission of the anemia if they could be absorbed [75, 187]; presumably a similar bacterial flora producing vitamin B$_{12}$ is present in the stools of vegans, who secrete intrinsic factor but still develop vitamin B$_{12}$ deficiency.

Since the small intestine provides the only physiologically significant absorptive surface for vitamin B$_{12}$, it is clear why any derangement in this portion of the alimentary canal may produce vitamin B$_{12}$ deficiency disease if the derangement is of sufficient chronicity so that the body stores of available vitamin B$_{12}$ are exhausted.

Study of individuals who had undergone total gastrectomy indicate that such stores become depleted to a sufficient extent to produce a macrocytosis in approximately one or two years, with anemia appearing in another one or two years, and a megaloblastic marrow shortly thereafter.[30] The major site of storage of vitamin B$_{12}$ appears to be the liver,[35, 188] in which the biologic half-life of vitamin B$_{12}$ is approximately a year.[37]

In most patients with a small intestinal disorder of sufficient degree to produce defective absorption of vitamin B$_{12}$, oral administration of supplementary intrinsic factor is not able to improve the absorption.[189-191]

It is not easy to predict the time of onset of overt clinical vitamin B$_{12}$ deficiency in any patient with an absorptive defect, because the amount of the body stores, the dietary intake, and the metabolic turnover of vitamin B$_{12}$ varies from person to person. In addition, failure to absorb vitamin B$_{12}$ is usually not absolute, and varies from time to time in the same individual.

1. Malabsorption Syndrome

"Malabsorption syndrome" is a term applied to a group of metabolic disorders in which multiple defects of intestinal absorption play a prominent part.[192-199, 199a]

a. *Primary*

Primary malabsorption syndrome includes those generalized absorption defects of unknown etiology in which varying degrees of atrophy of the intestinal villi are present.[200-205] The possible existence of receptors for intrinsic factor in the small intestine [111, 112, 206] suggests a direct relationship between the degree of damage of the intestinal villi (with concomitant reduction in number of receptors) and the degree of inability to absorb vitamin B_{12}. A similar relationship may exist for folic acid absorption. The variable degree and reversibility of the atrophy of the intestinal villi may explain in part the similar variable degree and reversibility of the absorptive defect for vitamin B_{12}.[190, 191, 207, 208]

Another factor which must be considered in evaluating the absorptive defect for vitamin B_{12}, in both primary and secondary malabsorption syndromes, is the dependence of intrinsic factor action on calcium.[112] Removal of calcium by fatty acids in the form of insoluble soaps may explain the poor vitamin B_{12} absorption in some patients with steatorrhea,[209] although in one series [158] of 10 such patients, peroral administration of 7 to 10 Gm. of calcium lactate had no significant effect on absorption of concurrently administered radio-B_{12}.

The various conditions forming the group characterized as the *primary malabsorption syndrome* are differentiated from each other on clinical grounds such as age, place of residence, severity, response to treatment, and reversibility of the disease.[199]

Although the primary malabsorption states frequently are accompanied by considerably impaired absorption of vitamin B_{12}, they are generally more intimately related to folic acid deficiency, and will be discussed further in that connection.

(1). *Tropical sprue.* This steatorrhea syndrome seen in the tropics is probably most often the result of prolonged dietary deficiency of folic acid.[210-212] The associated absorptive defect for vitamin B_{12} is sometimes correctible by maintaining the patient on adrenocorticotrophic hormone (ACTH) [213] or adrenocortical steroids.[207] The mechanism of this correction is unknown. Response of megaloblastic anemia to administration of adrenocortical steroids has been observed in some cases of adult coeliac disease and of pernicious anemia [214, 215]; here, too, the mechanism of action of the steroids in terms of vitamin B_{12} (or folic acid) absorption is unknown.

Permanent correction of the absorptive defect usually follows effective treatment of the folic acid deficiency, which results in regeneration [205] of the intestinal villi,[203] if the damage has not persisted for such a prolonged period as to be irreversible, and generally a complete recovery of the patient.[204, 216, 217]

For these reasons, and because tropical sprue does not respond to a gluten-free diet and often demonstrates a return of the folic acid excretion test to normal with treatment,[204] tropical sprue is considered here, as it is by many authorities,[193, 203, 204, 217, 218] to differ from nontropical sprue. In the latter condition, the villi do not regenerate,[203] actual cure does not occur,[219] the patient often responds to a gluten-free diet,[219, 219a] and the folic acid excretion test remains abnormal after treatment.[204] It should be noted, however, that some investigators believe that the dissimilarities are too superficial to warrant definition of tropical and nontropical sprue as separate entities.[220, 221]

(2). *Childhood coeliac disease; adult coeliac disease (idiopathic steatorrhea, nontropical sprue).* These conditions are believed to be the expression of the same basic defect at different ages.[204, 218, 222] The villous atrophy is irreversible,[203, 223] and cure is not yet possible.[219, 224, 225]

This entity is probably the final result of a hereditary constitutional defect in metabolism transmitted as a dominant trait of variable penetrance and expressivity.[204, 218, 226–229] It has been stated that "pernicious anemia is the final result of a genetically determined progressive atrophy of the chief cells of gastric mucosa, while coeliac disease and idiopathic steatorrhoea result from an analagous atrophy of the crypt cells of the intestinal mucosa." [203]

b. *Secondary*

Secondary malabsorption syndrome includes those clinical entities which produce gross pathologic alteration in the structure or function of the small intestine of sufficient degree and duration to result in deranged absorptive capacity. The degree of the derangement is a major factor in determining whether vitamin B_{12} (and folic acid) deficiency will be produced.

(1). *Regional ileitis.* Megaloblastic anemia is a not infrequent result of this condition,[230] which frequently produces grossly deficient vitamin B_{12} absorption. In one study, 42 patients out of 80 had low serum vitamin B_{12} levels, and the impaired absorption could almost always be restored to normal by steroid therapy.[229]

(2). *Strictures or anastomoses of the small bowel.* Megaloblastic anemia has been observed to follow the development of single or multiple small bowel strictures, usually in the ileum, and intestinal anastomoses.[231, 232] The latter have included entero-enterostomies, enterocolostomies, gastrojejunocolic fistulae, and gastrocolic fistulae.

Defective absorption of vitamin B_{12} or folic acid or both is demonstrable in a significant percentage of such patients.[221] However, in the majority of such patients, when macrocytic anemia develops it appears to be the result of intestinal stasis producing an abnormal bacterial flora and the blind loop syndrome, rather than a secondary malabsorption syndrome.[231, 233]

(3). *Intestinal resection.* Intestinal resections, as performed for jejunoileitis or superior mesenteric artery occlusions, may result in failure adequately to absorb vitamin B_{12}.[191, 234]

(4). *Malignancies and granulomatous lesions involving the small intestine.* Lymphosarcoma, reticulum cell sarcoma, lymphogranulomatosis, and intestinal lipodystrophy are among the conditions which may produce a malabsorption syndrome with compromise of vitamin B_{12} absorption to a variable degree.[235–238]

(5). *Other conditions characterized by chronically disturbed intestinal function.* Macrocytic anemia has been reported in such conditions associated with chronic intestinal dysfunction as chronic pancreatic disease,[239] chronic dysentery,[240] hypothyroidism,[157] and mesenteric vascular disease.[208] In the latter two conditions, resolution of the metabolic disorder and healing of the intestinal lesion respectively were associated with a return to normal of the intestinal absorption of vitamin B$_{12}$, which had been previously demonstrated to be greatly reduced. There is some evidence in rats that the absorptive mechanism in the ileum for vitamin B$_{12}$ is slowed down by hypothyroidism.[241] Decreased secretion of intrinsic factor may also occur with lack of thyroid hormone.

2. Specific Malabsorption for Vitamin B$_{12}$

a. *Due to Long Term Ingestion of Calcium-Chelating Agents*

The mechanism of intrinsic factor action in the intestine appears to be calcium-dependent.[111, 112, 206, 242] The amount of radioactive vitamin B$_{12}$ excreted in the urine of normal subjects during the course of a Schilling test after short term administration of calcium-chelating agents such as sodium phytate or ethylene-diamine-tetraacetate (EDTA) is considerably decreased.[206, 243] In some patients with steatorrhea, oral administration of calcium lactate increases the otherwise small amount of vitamin B$_{12}$ absorbed.[209] In most cases it has no effect, however.[158]

Five patients receiving orally administered sodium phytate for periods from 19 to 44 months as treatment for hypercalcuria associated with renal stones,[244] were investigated through the courtesy of Dr. P. H. Henneman. They were all found to have decreased serum vitamin B$_{12}$ levels, increasingly marked in direct proportion to the length of therapy, macroovalocytosis, an increased amount of hypersegmentation of the nuclei of the polymorphonuclear leukocytes, and diminished position and/or vibration sense in the toes.[206, 242]

Examination of the bone marrow morphology in each of these 5 patients revealed the presence of some intermediate megaloblasts and some large, but not quite giant, metamyelocytes.

The inference from these studies would seem to be that patients receiving prolonged oral therapy with oral calcium-chelating agents will eventually develop a full blown megaloblastic anemia due to vitamin B_{12} deficiency, if not prophylactically treated by injection of the vitamin at regular intervals. However, absorption of radioactive vitamin B_{12}, in 2 μg. doses, by the 5 patients on prolonged phytate therapy appeared to be normal.[206] Since it was not determined that the radioactivity absorbed was that of the vitamin B_{12}, rather than that of a breakdown product of the vitamin, and since other possibilities also could explain the discrepant results, further study is needed to determine clearly whether or not long term ingestion of calcium-chelating agents will sufficiently restrict B_{12} absorption eventually to cause full blown megaloblastic anemia. All the evidence, except for the normal absorption of radioactive vitamin B_{12}, suggests that overt megaloblastic anemia will in fact eventually develop in such cases.

b. *Due to Absence of Intestinal Receptors for Intrinsic Factor*

According to a recent hypothesis,[110–112] which coincides with the views of various workers,[113–115, 115a] receptors for intrinsic factor exist in the small intestine and play a vital role in the absorption of physiologic amounts of vitamin B_{12}. It would be logical to suspect that if such receptors exist, patients might be found who are unable to absorb vitamin B_{12} because of a congenital or acquired reduction or absence of these receptors, independent of any other absorptive defects.

In a search for such patients, the author has seen 7 individuals with megaloblastic anemia, serum vitamin B_{12} levels below 100 $\mu\mu$g./ml., inability to absorb a 2 μg. oral dose of radioactive vitamin B_{12} either alone or with added hog intrinsic factor concentrate, intrinsic factor secretion appearing to be normal as measured by in vitro "assay" of gastric juice, and no steatorrhea, diarrhea, or other signs or symptoms of malabsorption syndrome.

Two of these patients developed steatorrhea during fat balance studies, and were classified as cases of adult coeliac disease.

A third, B.C., a 70 year old woman of Puerto Rican origin, was extensively studied at the Mount Sinai Hospital. Examination included a full battery of studies for possible malabsorption of agents other than vitamin B$_{12}$ by Dr. D. Adlersberg's group. Glucose, fat, vitamin A and xylose tolerance tests, fat balance studies, gastrointestinal tract roentgenograms and fluoroscopy, plasma prothrombin, and serum calcium, phosphorus, alkaline phosphatase, and "folic acid" were all normal.

This woman was one of the patients we made available to Drs. Luhby, Cooperman, and Teller for their studies using their method of histidine loading[511]; they found "no biochemical folic acid deficiency" (as manifested by excretions of formiminoglutamic acid in the urine which were well within the normal range after many repeated histidine loading doses).

There was free acid in her gastric juice after, but not before, histamine stimulation. The only suggestion of an absorptive abnormality other than for vitamin B$_{12}$ was a low serum carotene level of 51 μg. per cent. This could have been explained on the basis of her poor diet,[602] but it could also be a reflection of an otherwise completely hidden malabsorption syndrome.

The fourth patient, M.C., was studied at the Mount Sinai Hospital almost exactly as patient B.C. (*vide supra*). This 71 year old woman of Puerto Rican origin had a serum carotene level of 43 μg. per cent and a serum "folic acid" level of 2.4 mμg./ml., indicative of folic acid depletion despite the absence of formiminoglutamic acid in her urine (l-histidine loading was not done in this case). All other studies yielded normal results. While her low serum carotene could be explained by her poor diet, it is harder to explain the low serum "folic acid" level. She is being further studied to delineate more clearly the condition. The present working diagnosis is malabsorption syndrome, but dietary folic acid deficiency plus a specific absorptive defect for vitamin B_{12} due to lack of intestinal receptors for intrinsic factor remains an alternate possibility.

The final 3 patients have been partially studied for absorptive defects other than for vitamin B_{12}, including three day fat balance studies, with no such defects found. This was also true of other cases alluded to in the literature.[173, 245]

One or more of the 5 above noted cases may eventually be definitively proved to have solely a specific absorptive defect for vitamin B_{12} due to a reduction or absence of intestinal receptors for intrinsic factor, or of whatever other small intestinal mechanism or mechanisms which may be involved in vitamin B_{12} absorption. In all of these 5 cases, repetitive studies at varying intervals of time are required to rule out an occult generalized malabsorption syndrome whose various other parameters may be only intermittently demonstrable. Other cases of possible specific malabsorption for vitamin B_{12} are being closely followed elsewhere.[245a]

At present it may be said that specific malabsorption for vitamin B_{12} does exist, but its existence as an entity independent of adult coeliac disease (and possibly other etiologic entities in the group of generalized malabsorption syndromes) cannot be considered proved until extensive longitudinal studies over a period of years have been carried out, or until jejunal biopsies are obtained.

It must be remembered that some patients with malabsorption syndrome may not demonstrate malabsorption for fats, even on serially repeated studies, and may show malabsorption only for glucose on one occasion, only for vitamin A on another occasion, etc.

Unfortunately, none of our five patients had jejunal biopsy. Demonstration of a normal jejunal mucosa in these individuals would effectively exclude idiopathic steatorrhea and help to establish definitively the diagnosis of specific malabsorption for vitamin B_{12}.

C. Competition for Vitamin B$_{12}$ by Intestinal Parasites or Bacteria

1. Fish Tapeworm (Diphyllobothrium Latum)

Next to addisonian pernicious anemia, fish tapeworm anemia is probably the most thoroughly investigated of all the vitamin B$_{12}$ deficiency states.[100] It has been directly demonstrated both in vitro [246] and in vivo [247] that the fish tapeworm competes directly with the intrinsic factor of the host for available vitamin B$_{12}$ in the intestine.[248]

The higher the parasite is located, the more likely it is to interfere with vitamin B$_{12}$ absorption,[247, 249] since the vitamin has less prolonged contact with the intestine, and therefore less chance of being absorbed, prior to being taken up by the tapeworm.

Other factors influencing the relative uptake of vitamin B$_{12}$ by the parasite as compared to the host are the number and size of the worms,[100, 247] the rapidity of growth and of egg production by the worms,[247] and the quantity of intrinsic factor produced by the host.[248] Vitamin B$_{12}$ bound to intrinsic factor is unavailable to the parasite,[246] but is available to the host.

Vitamin B$_{12}$ in high concentration appears to be an essential constituent of the fish tapeworm. The concentration of vitamin B$_{12}$ per gram of dried worm is from 1.33 to 3 μg., easily enough to provide treatment in pernicious anemia. Although the concentration of vitamin B$_{12}$ in Ascaris lumbricoides is of the same magnitude, vitamin B$_{12}$ deficiency has not with certainty been found in cases of infestation with this parasite, perhaps because of differences in quantity and biologic properties of these parasites as compared to the fish tapeworm. Other parasites, such as Taenia saginata, contain considerably less vitamin B$_{12}$ and do not appear capable of causing vitamin B$_{12}$ deficiency.[100]

2. Bacteria: The Blind Loop Syndrome [250]

Megaloblastic anemia may appear in association with the presence of a surgically created blind loop of intestine,[251] in the presence of the multiple small blind loops of massive small intestinal diverticulosis,[252] or with intestinal stricture or anastomosis.[231, 233] In such cases, impaired absorption of vitamin B_{12} has been repeatedly demonstrated.

The defective vitamin B_{12} absorption may be greatly improved during administration of one of the tetracycline group of antibiotics,[251, 252] but not by neomycin or sulfisoxazole.[233] The response to antibiotics, the avidity of certain strains of intestinal bacteria for vitamin B_{12},[253] and the evidence from autopsy studies [233] and animal experiments [254, 255] that an abnormal small intestinal bacterial flora proliferating in the stagnant loops of small intestine was an invariable occurrence when macrocytic anemia developed, all led to the concept that stasis of intestinal content, with abnormal bacterial growth, results in impaired absorption of vitamin B_{12}, and possibly of folic acid, possibly by diversion from the host to the bacteria.[256] In some cases the major deficiency may be of folic acid rather than vitamin B_{12}.[233]

While the mechanism of this phenomenon may be direct competition for available vitamin B_{12} and folic acid in the intestine by the bacteria and the host, this mechanism is not as clearly demonstrated in the blind loop syndrome as it is in fish tapeworm anemia. One bit of evidence suggesting a possible role for the tetracyclines other than destruction of abnormal intestinal flora, is a report of slow but definite remission of pernicious anemia on administration of chlortetracycline.[257] This may have been spontaneous remission, but more study of this phenomenon may be useful.

In certain megaloblastic anemias in Kenya, dramatic improvement has been reported after treatment with oral penicillin alone.[258] It was speculated that the high carbohydrate-low animal protein diet of these natives might produce an abnormal small bowel bacterial flora.

III. INADEQUATE UTILIZATION

A. Inability to Utilize Vitamin B_{12}

The existence of this entity has not yet been established with certainty. Cases of pernicious anemia have been reported in which the patients ceased to respond to parenteral vitamin B$_{12}$ therapy and showed a return to megaloblastic hematopoiesis after developing extensive gastric carcinoma.[43, 259, 260] The author has observed a possibly similar phenomenon in a 260 pound female patient with pernicious anemia in remission who developed carcinoma of the breast with extensive metastases to bones.[261] She went into hematologic relapse despite continuation of her maintenance dosage of 60 μg. of vitamin B$_{12}$ parenterally at monthly intervals. The patient died before it could be determined whether the hematologic picture could be improved by administration of larger amounts of vitamin B$_{12}$ or administration of folic acid; the serum vitamin B$_{12}$ level just prior to death was 620 $\mu\mu$g./ml. by L. Leishmanii assay (a normal result), but her red cell B$_{12}$ level was only 180 $\mu\mu$g./ml. (In the normal subject, serum and red cell vitamin B$_{12}$ levels are roughly the same.) It is not known whether the phenomenon of relapse despite continuation of the maintenance dosage of vitamin B$_{12}$ in these patients was a reflection of inability to utilize vitamin B$_{12}$, increased demand for the vitamin, or yet another cause, such as folic acid deficiency. In the light of present knowledge, the latter possibility seems most likely. (See section, "Parasitization of Folic Acid by Malignant Tissue," page 59.)

Recent experimental evidence in rats that vitamin B$_{12}$ may be a co-factor in amino acid incorporation into protein [262, 263] has been accompanied by demonstration of inhibition of protein biosynthesis by the anilide of the monocarboxylic acid of vitamin B$_{12}$, which seemed to function as an anti-vitamin B$_{12}$ in this reaction.[262]

Future studies using anti-vitamin B$_{12}$ agents as antimetabolites to reduce the speed of neoplastic growth in humans, much as the antifolic acid agents are now used, may produce clear-cut cases of inability to utilize vitamin B$_{12}$. Preliminary studies [206, 264, 265] suggest this possibility may soon be realized, with the use of altered vitamin B$_{12}$ molecules which may act by blocking the vitamin B$_{12}$ transport and storage systems, by competitive inhibition of vitamin B$_{12}$, or both.

B. Parasitization by Fetus

Serum vitamin B_{12} levels gradually decrease during pregnancy, and vitamin B_{12} levels of umbilical cord blood are invariably higher than those of the mother obtained at the same time.[266–269, 269a] Supraphysiologic (1000 μg.) oral doses of vitamin B_{12} may be absorbed at a greater than normal rate by pregnant women,[270] but depressed absorption of physiologic doses has been reported.[271] This depressed absorption may be due to decreased secretion of intrinsic factor; it is known that gastric secretion of acid and pepsin falls during pregnancy.[272, 273]

Despite the lowering during pregnancy, serum vitamin B_{12} levels generally remain within normal limits. This is not always true, however,[274, 275, 489b] Megaloblastic anemia rarely occurs during pregnancy when nutrition is adequate [273, 276]; when it occurs with poor nutrition, it is more frequently due to primary deficiency of folic acid than of vitamin B_{12}.[10, 277–281]

The combination of a marginal vitamin B_{12} intake and parasitization of available vitamin B_{12} by the fetus could lead to a vitamin B_{12} deficiency in the mother. Such a deficiency has not been frequently reported, but does occur.[274, 275, 489b]

C. Inability to Retain Absorbed Vitamin B_{12}

Most of the vitamin B_{12} in human serum is bound to serum proteins,[282] primarily to an alpha-1 globulin.[282, 283] It appears from studies in vitro that amounts of vitamin B_{12} in excess of physiologic serum levels may be bound to other fractions, including beta globulins.[284, 284a]

It is possible that deficiency or absence of the vitamin B_{12} binding protein in serum could lead to inability to retain vitamin B_{12}. A single case of macrocytic anemia with a defect in vitamin B_{12} binding has been reported.[285] That patient's macrocytic anemia could not be maintained in abeyance by 30 μg. of vitamin B_{12} intramuscularly at one to two week intervals, and intramuscular administration of 0.5 μg. of Co^{60}-labeled vitamin B_{12} resulted in the urinary excretion of 60 per cent of the administered dose within 24 hours. (Normal persons excreted 0 to 10 per cent under similar conditions.) After giving normal plasma, the urinary excretion of the same dose of labeled vitamin decreased to 24 per cent. Temporary remission could be produced by a single intramuscular dose of 90 μg. of vitamin B$_{12}$ or by the intravenous administration of 250 ml. of human plasma. The patient had unexplained unresponsiveness to weekly injections of crude liver extract for 18 years prior to demonstration of her response to normal plasma administration.

In a recent personal communication, Horrigan provided further information regarding the patient, including the following:

> Prior to treatment her serum vitamin B$_{12}$ level was only 52 μμg./ml. (E. gracilis assay, performed by A. Lear at Thorndike Memorial Laboratory), confirming the existence of vitamin B$_{12}$ deficiency. After three successive responses to plasma, the patient became refractory to it. Her vitamin B$_{12}$ requirement to maintain remission gradually rose to daily injections of 1,000 μg. Iron deficiency anemia developed. A bleeding hiatus hernia was found and operatively repaired. The patient died a month after the operation, after a few days of rapidly increasing icterus and terminal bleeding from all orifices. At postmortem examination the findings were: multiple endocrine tumors (chromophobe adenoma of pituitary, adenomatosis of parathyroids, islet cell tumors of pancreas, islet cell tumor of jejunum), cortical hyperplasia of adrenals, slight nephrocalcinosis and acute massive distention of intestine.

The exact mechanisms of her defect with respect to vitamin B$_{12}$ were never worked out. A possible relationship to an occult malabsorption syndrome or to one or more of her endocrine abnormalities was not demonstrated prior to her death. Study of other such cases, when found, may throw considerable light on the mechanism of vitamin B$_{12}$ binding, transport, and storage.

5 *Etiologic Classification of the Megaloblastic Anemias Due to Folic Acid Deficiency and Other Causes*

ETIOLOGIC CLASSIFICATION of the folic acid deficiency states has been hampered by a number of problems. The daily dietary requirement for folic acid is unknown.[286] Because of the efficacy of oral treatment of folic acid deficiency states, no extensive studies have been reported indicating the minimal parenteral maintenance dose for folic acid-deficient patients. Therefore no baseline has been established for studies relating to the possibly different requirement for folic acid of individuals with various forms of folic acid deficiency.

This is especially true of the folic acid deficiency states of pregnancy and infancy, where increased requirement for folic acid almost certainly exists, as a result of the increased metabolic load carried by the mother and the growth requirement of the infant.

Because of the simplicity of oral treatment with 5 to 15 mg. doses of folic acid in patients with intestinal malabsorption, very little information is available as to whether malabsorption is the cause or the effect of folic acid deficiency in these individuals. It is quite probable, for example, that the folic acid deficiency of many cases of tropical sprue is primarily due to an inadequate diet,[210] and that the folic acid deficiency itself produces intestinal malabsorption, diarrhea, and perpetuation of the deficiency due to the resulting impaired absorption of folic acid.

Determination of baseline blood levels of folic acid is considered valueless by most workers [287, 288]; the available evidence is that folic acid and the chemically well defined folic acid-active substances are not ordinarily present in human blood.[289]

Balance studies cannot be used to study the absorption of folic acid because fecal excretion considerably exceeds dietary intake of the vitamin, probably due to its synthesis by intestinal bacteria.[290]

In the light of present knowledge, no clear separation of the folic acid deficiency states caused by failure to ingest folic acid from those caused by failure to absorb the vitamin is possible. The general heading of "Nutritional Folic Acid Deficiency" will therefore be used to encompass those states characterized by variable degrees of inadequate intake and inadequate absorption of folic acid. The relative roles of inadequate diet and defective absorption in each condition will be indicated insofar as it is possible, but the reader must realize that future knowledge may necessitate revision of the relative significance attributed to these two factors in any given clinical state.

The recent demonstration that folic acid deficiency may be measured easily in man [489, 489a,489b] may prove a stepping stone on the road to solution of many of these problems.

I. NUTRITIONAL FOLIC ACID DEFICIENCY

A. Inadequate Diet

The daily dietary requirement of a normal man for folic acid is estimated to be less than one mg.[286, 291] The excellent hematologic response of some folic acid-deficient patients to parenteral administration of as little as 250 μg. daily [84] suggests that the daily requirement may be less than 0.25 mg. As stated above, more studies with parenteral administration of small doses of folic acid in folic acid-deficient patients are needed to delineate more clearly the minimal daily requirement for this vitamin.

The major dietary sources of folic acid are animal liver and kidney, and fresh green leafy (and nonleafy) vegetables.[292] Dried kidney beans, navy beans, and soy beans are also high in folic acid content, as are peanuts, almonds, coconuts, and some fresh fruits.

It should be noted that from 50 to 95 per cent of the folic acid content of foods may be lost in cooking [293]; losses may be especially great in canned foods.[294]

TABLES 1 AND 2 present the distribution of folic acid in foods,[295] and provide a useful reference when attempting to determine whether the diet of a given patient is deficient in folic acid. The values are for *fresh uncooked foods* only.

It should be remembered that most diets which are deficient in folic acid are also inadequate in vitamin B_{12}, though to a lesser degree. A striking exception to this rule is the folic acid deficiency associated with a milk diet. Milk of most kinds is uniquely low in folic acid but contains adequate quantities of vitamin B_{12}.[79, 296] An additional factor favoring general predominance of folic acid dietary deficiency is a possibly somewhat greater stability of vitamin B_{12} and greater retention in foods with cooking.

1. Megaloblastic Anemias in Infancy

Because of the low folic acid content of milk, infants subsisting entirely on milk may develop megaloblastic anemia.[297–300, 299a] Concomitant ascorbic acid deficiency can often be expected, especially when the infant is fed cow's milk, which even when undiluted contains only one quarter as much vitamin C as breast milk.[301] (See section, "Inadequate Utilization of Folic Acid due to Ascorbic Acid Deficiency," page 58.)

Evaporated milk,[292] dried milk, goat's milk, and breast milk [79, 296] all may provide inadequate quantities of folic acid. The megaloblastic anemia of infants fed goat's milk exclusively has been described as a separate entity, but this anemia shows the typical recovery pattern following folic acid therapy.[300]

Megaloblastic anemia following the ingestion of a diet consisting almost exclusively of milk has been reported in adults who were emotionally disturbed (usually depressed),

TABLE 1.—*Folic Acid (PGA-Pteroylglutamic Acid) Content of Foods*

Food	Moisture, %	Total PGA content, fresh basis, γ/g.
Meats and Eggs		
Beef, round steak	70	0.06–0.14
Beef, heart	76	0.03
Beef, kidney	76	0.58
Beef, sweetbreads	78	0.23
Beef, liver	68	2.9
Lamb, stew meat	59	0.03
Lamb, liver	69	2.76
Pork, loin	66	0.03
Pork, liver	68	2.2
Pork, ham (smoked)	67	0.10
Chicken, dark meat	77	0.03
Chicken, white meat	77	0.03
Chicken, liver	72	3.77
Eggs, whole	74	0.03–0.08
Egg white	87	0.004
Egg yolk	50	0.13
Nuts		
Peanuts	1	0.51
Almonds	4	0.45
Coconuts	44	0.27
Vegetables, fresh		
Asparagus	93	0.89–1.42
Beans, lima	70	0.10–0.40
Beans, green snap	90	0.14–0.41
Beets	86	0.10–0.15
Broccoli	91	0.24–0.35
Brussels sprouts	84	0.20–0.34
Cabbage	92	0.11–0.75
Carrots	88	0.07–0.15
Cauliflower	91	0.17–0.29
Corn, sweet	64–81	0.09–0.70
Cucumbers	96	0.97–2.07
Greens, beet	90	0.31–0.39
Greens, spinach	92	0.48–1.15
Lettuce	96	0.03–0.54
Peas, fresh	76	0.12–0.35
Peppers, green	94	0.04–0.09
Potatoes, peeled	80	0.04–0.06
Potatoes, peel	79	0.08–0.20
Pumpkin	92	0.05–0.10
Sweet potatoes	70	0.05–0.19
Tomatoes	92–94	0.02–0.15

From STOKSTAD, E. L. R.: Pteroylglutamic acid. VIII. Occurrence in foods. *In* Sebrell, W. H., Jr., and Harris, R. S.: The Vitamins. New York, Academic Press, 1954, vol. 3.

TABLE 2.—*Folic Acid (PGA-Pteroylglutamic Acid) Content of Foods*

Food	Moisture, %	Total PGA content, fresh basis, γ/g.
Vegetables, dried		
Beans, kidney	9	1.90
Beans, navy	11	1.28
Beans, soybeans	8	2.08
Peas, green split	9	0.24
Peas, yellow split	—	0.24
Fruits, fresh		
Apple, whole	84	0.04
Apricots	87	0.30
Bananas	73	0.35
Berries, blackberries	84	0.39–1.15
Berries, cranberries	88	0.13
Berries, strawberries	91	0.60
Cantaloupes	91	0.47–0.88
Cherries	80	0.30
Grapefruit	89	0.24
Grapes	80	0.20–0.29
Lemons	91	0.87
Oranges	86	0.28–0.40
Orange juice	87	0.36
Peaches	88	0.08–0.20
Pears	85	0.11–0.16
Fruits, dried		
Apricots	27	0.06
Peaches	25	0.07
Prunes	27	0.07
Raisins, seedless	17	0.13
Cereals and grains		
Barley	11	0.45
Corn, yellow	11	0.26
Oats	11	0.26
Rice, brown	5	0.12–0.35
Rice, milled	5	0.15
Sorghum grain		
White kafir	11	0.21
Yellow milo	10	0.24
Wheat	8.5–10.6	0.34–0.45
Dairy Products		
Buttermilk	88	0.11
Evaporated	73	0.07
Non-fat, dry	2.2	0.02
Cheese, Cheddar	34	0.19–0.29
Cheese, cottage	73–77	0.92

From STOKSTAD, E. L. R.: Pteroylglutamic acid. VIII. Occurrence in foods. *In* Sebrell, W. H., Jr., and Harris, R. S.: The Vitamins. New York, Academic Press, 1954, vol. 3.

and in adults in whom full-mouth dental extractions led to substitution of milk for all solid food.[302]

Infants with kwashiorkor or other debilitating conditions occasionally manifest a megaloblastic anemia. In such cases there are so many deficiencies (often including vitamin B_{12} deficiency) that it is difficult to assign a predominant role in the development of megaloblastosis to any one of them,[303] although treatment with folic acid usually is required and produces a reticulocytosis.[304, 305] The one four year old boy with kwashiorkor recently seen at The Mount Sinai Hospital had a megaloblastic anemia, with a serum vitamin B_{12} level of 52 $\mu\mu$g./ml., a serum "folic acid" level of 2.7 mμg./ml., and a serum iron level of 45 μg./ml. The iron deficiency had a moderate "masking" effect on the erythrocyte component of the megaloblastic picture due to the B_{12} and folic acid deficiencies.

Remission of megaloblastic anemia in infancy has occurred following vitamin B_{12} administration [306] perhaps due in the majority of cases to mobilization of residual stores of folic acid. Failure of response to vitamin B_{12} is frequent,[299, 307] but failures of response to folic acid therapy occasionally supplemented with ascorbic acid are relatively rare. It must be concluded that in most instances megaloblastic anemia in infancy is caused primarily by deficiency of folic acid. However, neurologic damage has been observed frequently enough, especially by European workers [307, 307a] so that concomitant or even primary vitamin B_{12} deficiency must always be looked for. The term, "megaloblastic anemia of infancy," should be discarded. It implies an etiologic unity which does not exist.

2. Megaloblastic Anemias in Pregnancy and Puerperium

The great majority of cases of megaloblastic anemia in pregnancy has been in women ingesting diets inadequate in folic acid content,[308] and often wholly inadequate, especially in meat content.[273] This inadequacy is accentuated by the increased requirement for folic acid during pregnancy,[309] especially during the last two months, when the fetal requirement for this vitamin may be maximal,[304] and overt folic acid deficiency appears.

While most cases of megaloblastic anemia in pregnancy and puerperium appear to result primarily from folic acid deficiency, some cases have superimposed vitamin B_{12} deficiency, or suffer from primary deficiency of vitamin B_{12}.[274, 275, 489b] Such deficiency may develop from the combination of a marginal diet, depressed absorption associated with pregancy,[271] with folic acid deficiency, and parasitization of the mother's vitamin B_{12} by the fetus. (See section, "Parasitization of Vitamin B_{12} by Fetus," page 42.)

The term, "megaloblastic anemia of pregnancy," implies an etiologic unity which does not exist, and should be discarded. A more accurate designation would be "megaloblastic anemia in pregnancy, due to folic acid deficiency and/or vitamin B_{12} deficiency caused by . . . (state specific cause or causes, such as poor diet)."

Careful search for early signs of megaloblastic anemia in the peripheral blood smears of all women admitted to hospital for delivery might reveal the incidence of megaloblastic anemia in pregnancy to be as high as 1 in every 39 patients in temperate zones,[273] or even higher. The incidence in the tropics is still higher.

Some cases have been reported in the presence of a presumably excellent diet and no known gastrointestinal disturbance.[310] However, such cases responded to folic acid therapy, thus leaving open the question as to etiology.

It is undecided as to whether impaired absorption of folic acid occurs during pregnancy. Girdwood[311] found no evidence for inadequate absorption, but more recent work[312] indicates that absorption of folic acid may be impaired in pregnant women.[304, 312]

The onset of megaloblastic anemia in pregnancy usually occurs in the last trimester, and sometimes in the puerperium.[313, 313a] Remission may appear spontaneously when the pregnancy terminates, but relapse may occur with a subsequent pregnancy or in the absence of another pregnancy.[276]

In the tropics, megaloblastic anemia of pregnancy may respond partially or completely to vitamin B_{12} alone.[277, 313–317] In temperate zones this may occur,[317] but is much less common, probably because general dietary deficiency stemming from economic and religious reasons with inadequacies of folic acid, vitamin B_{12}, and protein is much more common in tropical countries.[318]

Large doses of vitamin B_{12} often produce hematologic improvement.[319, 320] This may be due to a "mass action" effect of such doses, with mobilization of residual stores of folic acid. Such an effect is suggested by the fact that while vitamin B_{12} may induce a temporary remission, the end result of such therapy is disappointing in many cases if it is not supplemented with folic acid.[321] In some cases, of course, primary vitamin B_{12} deficiency may exist.

3. Nutritional Megaloblastic Anemia (Tropical and Nontropical Macrocytic Anemia)

Gross dietary deficiency resulting from poverty, ignorance, or religious tenets is widespread throughout the world, and especially in tropical areas. Such deficiency often encompasses a lack of animal protein and of fresh green vegetables.[6, 322] It therefore results in variable degrees of folic acid and vitamin B_{12} deficiency, in addition to deficiency of iron and sometimes of protein, as well.[7]

Many patients with nutritional megaloblastic anemia respond partially or completely to vitamin B_{12}.[277, 314–316, 323, 324] Slow and suboptimal responses are frequent, even with large doses of vitamin B_{12}.

On the other hand, a uniformly excellent response follows folic acid administration.[8, 211, 325–328]

Subnormal serum vitamin B_{12} levels have been reported in some cases of nutritional megaloblastic anemia,[10, 329, 330] but even in such cases folic acid was usually required in addition to vitamin B_{12} in order to obtain complete response to treatment.

Therefore, the megaloblastic anemia resulting from inadequate diets may be considered in almost all cases to be primarily a consequence of folic acid deficiency. In the production of these megaloblastic anemias, it is not yet determined whether the major role is played by a relatively greater deficiency of folic acid than of vitamin B_{12} in the diet, or relatively greater body stores and slower utilization of vitamin B_{12}. The author favors the latter possibility in the New York area because most of the patients with nutritional megaloblastic anemia of which he has personal knowledge were ingesting diets grossly inadequate in both vitamin B_{12} and folic acid, and yet they had normal serum vitamin B_{12} levels despite low serum "folic acid" levels.

4. Cirrhosis Associated with Chronic Alcoholism

Megaloblastic bone marrow pictures were observed in 4 of a group of 16 patients with macrocytic anemia associated with hepatic cirrhosis and chronic alcoholism.[84] In the patients with megaloblastic anemia demonstrable histologically, folic acid deficiency was proved by observation of subnormal daily urinary excretion of folic acid, failure to excrete administered folic acid promptly, and striking clinical and hematologic response to oral administration of 1350 μg. of conjugated folic acid plus 150 μg. of free folic acid daily.

The evidence suggested that folic acid deficiency developed in these patients through a combination of marginal or inadequate dietary intake plus a possible increased requirement for folic acid. While no evidence of folic acid deficiency was found in the 12 patients with macrocytic anemia *without* megaloblastic marrows, the possibility of incipient folic acid deficiency in those cases was not completely ruled out.

Further exploration of the etiology of the macrocytic anemias so often associated with hepatic disease is needed.[13a] Our own experience with patients with cirrhosis and macrocytic anemia would suggest that folic acid deficiency is usually present, manifested by low serum "folic acid" levels, regardless of whether the bone marrow morphology is clearly megaloblastic or appears to be normoblastic. In these latter patients, an Arneth count usually reveals a definite "shift to the right," as expected in early megaloblastic anemia.

B. Defective Absorption

As was stated in the discussion of the vitamin B_{12} deficiency states associated with small intestinal disorders (*vide supra*), variable degrees of reduced absorption of folic acid and of vitamin B_{12} may occur with any structural or functional disorder of the small intestine. If the disorder is chronic, clinically overt deficiency may eventually occur. Similar deficiency may occur in the presence of an abnormal intestinal flora, usually resulting from stagnation of intestinal contents (the blind loop syndrome). It is possible to infer that folic acid is absorbed primarily from the jejunum. Patients who have had large amounts of ileum resected may retain normal serum "folic acid" levels even a decade after the resection.[489b] Patients with idiopathic steatorrhea have lost much of their jejunal absorptive surface, but still may have normal ileal mucosa.[330a] Such patients invariably have low serum "folic acid" levels, and the levels may not rise to normal even after prolonged therapy with steroids or gluten-free diets.[489b, 512]

1. Malabsorption Syndrome

a. *Primary*

(1). *Tropical sprue.* Nearly all cases of tropical sprue appear to be closely related to deficiency of folic acid. Treatment with folic acid not only converts the hematologic picture to normal, but also brings about subsidence of the anorexia, diarrhea, steatorrhea, and other clinical signs and symptoms of tropical sprue.[331–335]

It is probable that the malabsorption syndrome of tropical sprue, with its accompanying defective absorption of folic acid,[312, 336] is the end result of dietary deficiency of folic acid, and should be classed as a *pseudo primary* malabsorption syndrome resulting from dietary deficiency of folic acid. Such dietary deficiency has been observed to be a significant factor in the pathogenesis of the disorder.[210–212]

Clear delineation of the pathogenesis has been confused by the demonstration of impaired absorption of folic acid in tropical sprue,[312, 336] and of return to normal folic acid absorption following the administration of a course of antibiotics.[312] The latter observation suggests the possibility that changes in the bacterial flora of the intestine, perhaps related to diet,[258] may be intimately involved in the development of the folic acid deficiency state.

Delineation of the etiology of tropical sprue has been further confused by including in this category individuals with non-tropical sprue who happened to be in the tropics.[218] Unlike in nontropical sprue, the associated atrophy of the intestinal villi in tropical sprue often disappears on treatment,[203] and complete recovery of the patient is very frequent.[216, 217, 331–335]

(2). *Childhood and adult coeliac disease (idiopathic steator-rhea, nontropical sprue).* Unlike tropical sprue, the existence of which as a clear-cut condition independent of dietary folic acid deficiency is in doubt, the existence of childhood and adult coeliac disease as a single etiologic entity is becoming firmly established.[204, 222, 226–228, 337] Its existence as a hereditary constitutional defect in metabolism associated with irreversible atrophy of the small intestinal villi has been discussed in connection with the development in this condition of a secondary absorptive defect for vitamin B_{12}.

It is probable that the metabolic defect is enzymatic and associated with folic acid metabolism,[204] but it is undetermined whether the primary defect is in the transport of folic acid or its conjugates across the intestinal barrier or in their utilization after absorption. Poor transport across the intestinal mucosa is suggested by the low fasting serum "folic acid" levels of patients with idiopathic steatorrhea, before *and after* years of treatment with steroids or a gluten-free diet.

In this connection, determination of the fasting serum "folic acid" level in the relatives of patients with idiopathic steatorrhea may prove fruitful. Such a study might uncover a number of persons with latent disease manifested only by a serum "folic acid" level slightly below normal, and thereby provide information of value in further delineating the genetic pattern of idiopathic steatorrhea.

The anemia of childhood coeliac disease is usually microcytic and hypochromic, while that in the adult expression of the disorder is macrocytic.[218, 337, 338] A rare case of macrocytic anemia may be found in childhood coeliac disease.[339]

The megaloblastic anemia which occurs in the adult form of coeliac disease generally responds to folic acid administration,[340] and incompletely or not at all to vitamin B_{12}.[341-343] Unlike in tropical sprue, however, in nontropical sprue treatment with folic acid is not usually associated with a general improvement of symptoms and signs other than those due to the megaloblastic anemia, and not infrequently some anemia and macrocytosis may persist.[344-348] When this occurs, associated vitamin B_{12} deficiency may be found.

b. *Secondary*

Folic acid deficiency is rare in those conditions producing a secondary malabsorption syndrome without the growth of an abnormal intestinal bacterial flora (such as may accompany intestinal strictures and anastomoses). The latter conditions will be discussed below.

C. Competition for Folic Acid by Intestinal Bacteria: The Blind Loop Syndrome

As stated in the discussion of this syndrome under the heading of the vitamin B_{12} deficiency states, the major deficiency in any given case of blind loop syndrome may be of either folic acid or vitamin B_{12}.

Cases have been described in which the associated megaloblastic anemia failed to respond to vitamin B_{12} but was adequately treated with folic acid.[256] The reverse situation has also been documented.[233]

It may be that the type of deficiency which predominates will depend on the relative requirement and avidity for folic acid and vitamin B_{12} of the abnormal bacterial intestinal flora associated with the particular case of blind loop syndrome.

II. INADEQUATE UTILIZATION OF FOLIC ACID

A. Inability to Utilize

1. Due to Administration of Folic Acid Antagonists

Agents such as 4-aminopteroyl glutamic acid (Aminopterin), by blocking the utilization of folic acid, can produce a megaloblastic anemia.[349, 384]

This anemia is not reversible by folic acid administration, since 4-amino analogs of folic acid not only compete with folinic acid but also block the conversion of folic acid to folinic acid.[350] It may be reversed by administration of citrovorum factor (folinic acid), which bypasses the block.[350, 351]

2. Due to Administration of Anticonvulsants or Pyrimethamine

The appearance of megaloblastic anemia in patients being treated for prolonged periods of time with anticonvulsant drugs has been reported with increasing frequency.[352, 353] Drugs involved include Dilantin (Phenytoin)(diphenylhydantoin sodium),[354–357] Primidone (Mysoline)(5-phenyl-5-ethyl-hexahydro-pyrimidine-4,6-dione),[358–360] Rutonal (methophenobarbital),[361] and occasionally other barbiturates, including Amytal (amylobarbitone) and Seconal (quinalbarbitone).[353, 362] Megaloblastic anemia has not yet been reported following the use of phenobarbital, probably because of the low dose of this agent usually administered.[361]

The megaloblastic anemia which occurs responds either to withdrawal of the anticonvulsant[363] or to administration of folic acid,[353–359] and weakly or not at all to vitamin B_{12}, except in very large doses.[352–359, 364]

The absorption and tissue stores of folic acid in these patients appear to be normal in some, but in others the clearance of intravenously injected folic acid was abnormally rapid,[304, 365] suggesting a possible deficiency in tissue stores of the vitamin. Other interpretations of this finding are possible, and it is believed at present that the anticonvulsants must in some manner interfere in the utilization of folic acid. It is possible they act in part by competing with folic acid for intestinal absorption.

The chemical structure of the anticonvulsants resembles the pteridine ring system of folic acid, with the pyrazine ring open and partly degraded. They also resemble, therefore, the pyrimidines involved in nucleoprotein synthesis, and it is possible they may interfere with pyrimidine utilization as well as folic acid utilization, and may produce a megaloblastic anemia in part by blocking pyrimidine incorporation into nucleoproteins.

The same may be true of pyrimethamine (Daraprim), a substituted pyrimidine (2,4-diamino-5-p-chlorphenyl-6-ethylpyrimidine) [366] used as an antimalarial drug. In large doses this agent can produce a megaloblastic anemia, which rapidly clears when the drug is withdrawn.[367, 368] The antimicrobial action of pyrimethamine for Streptococcus faecalis is blocked by either large amounts of folic acid or small amounts of folinic acid,[369] and its toxic effect on the growing rat is alleviated by folinic acid, but not by folic acid.[370] Thus, while structurally pyrimethamine is more closely related to thymine than to folic acid, existing evidence suggests it is more an antifolic acid than an antithymine.[371]

Serum vitamin B_{12} levels have usually been reported to be normal in cases of megaloblastic anemia due to anticonvulsant therapy,[353] but low levels were found in 2 cases.[353, 372] In one of these cases the low serum level of vitamin B_{12} was observed during folic acid therapy.[353] Generally, vitamin B_{12} deficiency is probably not a phenomenon of significance in the megaloblastic anemias resulting from anticonvulsant therapy.

A 63 year old man who had been taking Dilantin for 15 years was seen at the Mount Sinai Hospital with a megaloblastic anemia. His serum "folic acid" level was normal, but his serum vitamin B_{12} level was 32 $\mu\mu$g./ml. (E. Gracilis assay). In vitro "assay" of his gastric juice revealed no intrinsic factor, and Glass and Schilling testing revealed inability to absorb vitamin B_{12} correctible with orally administered intrinsic factor concentrate. The patient was thus revealed as a person with pernicious anemia. The Dilantin was a "red herring" in his case, revealing the necessity of careful work-up for other possibilities even when a seemingly obvious explanation for megaloblastic anemia presented itself.

3. Due to Ascorbic Acid Deficiency

There is evidence that ascorbic acid is involved in augmenting the conversion of folic acid to a metabolically more active form.[373, 374] A few cases of megaloblastic anemia appearing in patients with scurvy and cleared by treatment with ascorbic acid have been reported.[375-377]

However, the anemia associated with scurvy is usually normocytic,[378] and even in severe scurvy anemia may not occur at all.[375, 376, 378, 379] For these reasons, plus the fact that it has not been possible to produce anemia in man by experimental ascorbic acid deprivation,[380, 381] it is probable that megaloblastic anemia appears in ascorbic acid deficiency states only in the presence of an associated deficiency in the supply or metabolism of folic acid.[377]

Dietary deficiency of both ascorbic and folic acids has been implicated in the causation of the megaloblastic anemias of infancy.[298, 299, 382, 383] (See section, "Megaloblastic Anemias in Infancy," page 46.)

B. Parasitization

1. By Fetus

It was pointed out in the discussion of megaloblastic anemia in pregnancy that the majority of patients were ingesting a diet inadequate in folic acid content. The folic acid requirement of the rapidly growing fetus probably results in removal of a significant portion of the marginal amount of folic acid absorbed,[309] and overt folic acid deficiency with megaloblastic anemia is the result. The serum "folic acid" levels of newborns are almost invariably much higher than the levels in their mother's serum.[269a]

The low serum "folic acid" levels of women in the latter half of pregnancy after an oral dose of folic acid have been interpreted as due to impaired absorption of the vitamin.[312] An alternative explanation may be rapid uptake by the fetus, with the result that measurable serum levels in the mother are low.

2. By Malignant Tissue? (See Chapter 5, Other Causes)

A megaloblastic bone marrow picture has been observed in association with various malignant diseases.[2, 384-387] It may be particularly prominent in erythremic myelosis (DiGuglielmo's disease)[388-390] and erythroleukemia (the DiGuglielmo syndrome)[22, 388-390] and in acute leukemia, usually of the aleukemic type presenting as a refractory macrocytic anemia.[2, 47, 259, 384, 391-396] It is also not uncommon in polycythemia vera.[397]

An explanation for the megaloblastic marrow picture associated with widespread malignant disease was speculatively derived from the observations that in such disease there is a markedly reduced output of a test dose of folic acid,[311] and rapid clearance of an intravenous dose of this vitamin.[304] It was suggested that the reduced output in the urine was a result of utilization of folic acid at a rapid rate by rapidly growing neoplastic tissue. Such utilization could produce depletion of the body stores of folic acid, or perhaps just local depletion at the bone marrow level, especially if the diet contained only a marginal quantity of the vitamin, and megaloblastic anemia would then appear. Serum "folic acid" is sometimes low with widespread malignant disease.[489b]

It is also possible that the marrow cells may be unable to capture or utilize folic acid or vitamin B_{12} adequately in the presence of some malignancies.[396]

III. ACHRESTIC ANEMIA
(IDIOPATHIC REFRACTORY MEGALOBLASTIC ANEMIA)

"Achrestic anemia" and "idiopathic refractory megaloblastic anemia" are terms coined to classify those cases of megaloblastic anemia which did not seem to fit into any other category or to respond to liver therapy.[398, 399]

In some of these cases, megaloblastosis disappears when folic acid therapy is administered, leaving a hyperplastic bone marrow and a refractory normoblastic anemia. The megaloblastosis appeared to be a consequence of excessive utilization of folic acid by the hyperplastic bone marrow.[400]

The majority of these cases have responded to folic acid or liver extract, and it is probable that with the currently available clinical and laboratory procedures most of these cases, insofar as megaloblastic picture is concerned, will be classified among the folic acid deficiency states.[259] A few may be among the vitamin B_{12} deficiency conditions, and the very few which do not respond to either vitamin B_{12} or folic acid [401, 401a, 401b, 415] may be due to other possible causes of interference with nucleoprotein synthesis, such as those discussed in the next section.

OTHER CAUSES

In CHAPTER 3, "The Biochemical Basis of Megaloblastic Hematopoiesis," it was pointed out that the megaloblast is the product of interference with nucleoprotein metabolism. This interference may be caused either by direct inhibition or by depletion of the enzyme systems and building blocks necessary for nucleoprotein synthesis.

Although depletion of vitamin B_{12} or of folic acid is the cause of the overwhelming majority of megaloblastic anemias, such depletion has not as yet been generally considered to be present in some conditions which are occasionally accompanied by megaloblastic bone marrow pictures.

These conditions may be broadly characterized as associated with inhibition or depletion of the bone marrow.[2] They include agranulocytosis,[402, 403] myelofibrosis,[404] tuberculosis,[405, 405a] leishmaniasis,[406] sepsis,[407] hemochromatosis,[408, 409] radiation injury,[407] and various severe anemias, especially when associated with hemolysis.[410–412, 413a]

Future study may relate many of the megaloblastic cell

pictures associated with depletion of the bone marrow to deficiency of folic acid or vitamin B_{12}, in some cases with such deficiency only manifest at the bone marrow level, caused by inadequate or rapid utilization of these vitamins. Excessively rapid clearance of an intravenously administered dose of folic acid has been demonstrated in 5 cases of chronic myelofibrosis 1 of which had megaloblastic erythropoiesis which became normoblastic after oral folic acid therapy.[304] Rapid clearance of intravenously administered folic acid also occurs in hemolytic anemia.[304] Even in the absence of an overtly megaloblastic bone marrow in hemolytic anemia, folic acid in pharmacologic doses may produce a reticulocytosis.[413]

The logical belief that megaloblastic anemia in association with various hemolytic anemias may be the result of an increased utilization of folic acid in the presence of accelerated hematopoiesis is becoming increasingly popular.[413a]

Megaloblastic anemia associated with hemochromatosis has been demonstrated to respond to vitamin B_{12} and folic acid administration.[408, 414] There is evidence that some cases may result from a primary deficiency of vitamin B_6,[415, 416] but in only 1 case so far has this relationship been convincingly reported.

Direct interference with nucleoprotein synthesis may play a role in some cases of megaloblastic anemia associated with what appears to be inhibition of the bone marrow, such as agranulocytosis. Here, too, however, the possibility of folic acid deficiency must not be overlooked.

Aplastic anemia is frequently associated with macrocytosis, sometimes partly explainable by reticulocytosis, since reticulocytes are large red cells.[417] Some cases of aplastic anemia and of aregenerative anemia limited to the red cell series may be due to total bone marrow exhaustion as the end result of prolonged deprivation of vitamin B_{12} (or folic acid), which may have passed through a megaloblastic stage before eventuating in a hypocellular, nonmegaloblastic bone marrow.[418, 418a] Such a marrow may be capable of only a slow response, if any, to long term administration of vitamin B_{12} and folic acid. Widespread aplasia of the bone marrow as a terminal event was a common finding at autopsy of patients with pernicious anemia in the years prior to the discovery of liver therapy.[419]

A rare patient with megaloblastic anemia may have an esoteric defect along the synthetic pathway leading to nucleoprotein formation. One such patient was an infant with a refractory megaloblastic anemia associated with orotic acid excretion.[401b] The anemia responded only to steroids and a concentrated yeast extract containing a mixture of uridylic and cytidylic acids. The infant was believed to be unable to synthesize pyrimidine nucleotides adequately due to a block at the stage of conversion of orotic acid to orotidylic acid. It is unknown whether the infant might have been able to effect this conversion with the aid of folinic acid or of one of the B_{12} co-enzymes, which have been suggested [419a] possibly to be the main forms in which vitamin B_{12} is catalytically active in the enzymatic reactions of living cells. It has been suggested that conditions may exist in which, because of a block in the conversion of vitamin to co-enzyme, only the latter may have therapeutic value.[419a]

The subject of possible enzymatic defects in nucleoprotein synthesis in man, related or unrelated to defects in conversion of folic acid, folinic acid or vitamin B_{12} to catalytically active forms, is just beginning to be explored. Careful study of all patients with "refractory megaloblastic anemia," with the aid of a biochemical orientation, will undoubtedly uncover many exotic defects in the future.

The megaloblastic anemia picture sometimes seen in association with various widespread malignant diseases has been discussed in the section, "Parasitization of Folic Acid by Malignant Tissue." Future studies may well require reclassification of some or all of the megaloblastic anemias and megaloblastic bone marrow pictures associated with malignant disease into entirely different etiologic categories. At present, knowledge is too limited to permit definitive classification.

6 *Clinical Picture*

A CENTURY AGO, Addison described the clinical picture in pernicious anemia.[98] This description, which we now know may fit equally well an advanced case of any of the vitamin B_{12} deficiency states, and in most respects fits the folic acid deficiency states as well, has not been improved upon. Addison wrote in 1855:

The countenance gets pale, the whites of the eyes become pearly, *the general frame flabby rather than wasted;* the pulse perhaps large but remarkably soft and compressible, and occasionally with a slight jerk, especially under the slightest excitement. There is an increasing indisposition to exertion with an uncomfortable feeling of faintness or breathlessness on attempting it; the heart is readily made to palpitate; the whole surface presents a blanched, smooth and waxy appearance; the lips, gums and tongue seem bloodless; *the flabbiness of the solids increases;* the appetite fails, extreme languor and faintness supervene, breathlessness and palpitation being produced by the most trifling exertion or emotion; some slight edema is probably perceived about the ankles. The debility becomes extreme; the patient can no longer arise from his bed; *the mind occasionally wanders;* he falls into a prostrate and half torpid state, and at length expires. *Nevertheless, to the very last, and after a sickness of perhaps several months' duration, the bulkiness of the general frame and the obesity often present a most striking contrast* to the failure and exhaustion observable in every other respect.

The only parts of Addison's classic description which do not always fit the folic acid deficiency states as generally as those due to vitamin B_{12} deficiency have been italicized. While nervous instability may occur in folic acid deficiency, cerebral or other neurologic manifestations as a direct result of the deficiency have only been documented with lack of vitamin B_{12}.[33] The neurologic signs and symptoms which may be seen frequently in the malabsorption syndrome are probably not due to the folic acid deficiency, but rather to vitamin B_{12} deficiency.[420] Subnormal serum vitamin B_{12} levels (usually below 50 μg./ml.) were observed in every case of malabsorption syndrome with neurologic signs or symptoms seen by the author.

The other feature of Addison's description which is peculiar to vitamin B_{12} deficiency is persistence of bulkiness of the frame and obesity. In the folic acid deficiency states, perhaps because they are so often accompanied by many other deficiencies, emaciation is more usual.[421]

It is generally believed that nervous system involvement only occurs with vitamin B_{12} deficiency, and not with folic acid deficiency alone.[33, 420, 422] It has been suggested that this may be due to a requirement of the nervous system for vitamin B_{12} but not for folic acid.[423] Intensive protein synthesis is required to maintain the integrity of axons.[424–426] Protein synthesis is dependent on adequate production of RNA,[427] which in turn is influenced considerably by vitamin B_{12},[425, 426, 428, 429] and perhaps slightly less by folic acid.[430]

Folic acid appears to be involved intimately in DNA synthesis,[430, 431] and only indirectly in protein synthesis. These findings, plus recent evidence suggesting the possibility that vitamin B_{12} may be involved in the enzymatic incorporation of amino acids into proteins,[262, 432, 433] may help explain why nervous system damage occurs only in the presence of vitamin B_{12} deficiency, and not in the presence of folic acid deficiency alone. However, it should be noted that the direct involvement of vitamin B_{12} in protein synthesis has been questioned,[434, 435] and the mechanism whereby only vitamin B_{12} but not folic acid deficiency leads to nervous system damage remains a subject for much more study.

Another subject for future study is the possibility that vitamin B_{12} deficiency may result in inadequate synthesis of the lipoid moiety of the lipoproteins, which are normally present in high concentrations in erythrocyte envelopes and the myelin sheaths in both the central and peripheral nervous system.[425, 436] Inadequate maintenance of the myelin sheaths due to vitamin B_{12} deficiency but not folic acid deficiency is an attractive possible explanation for the neurologic damage associated with the former condition but not the latter.

The classic association of subacute combined degeneration (combined-system disease, posterolateral sclerosis, funicular degeneration) with vitamin B_{12} deficiency is well known.[437, 438] It should be noted, however, that the disease usually starts insidiously and not subacutely; combined lesions are often absent;

and lesions of the peripheral nerves occur much more frequently and much earlier than lesions of the central nervous system.[420, 439–441]

The use of the term "subacute combined degeneration" to include all of those changes in the nervous system which may occur as a result of vitamin B_{12} deficiency should probably be discontinued.[420, 442] The nervous system changes would be more accurately described by direct reference to the actual involvement (i.e., "peripheral nerve, spinal cord, or cerebral damage due to vitamin B_{12} deficiency," [33, 442]) or, in general terms, "vitamin B_{12} neuropathy." [420]

Paresthesia, especially numbness and tingling in the hands and feet, is the most frequent neurologic symptom of vitamin B_{12} deficiency.[13, 439, 443] Not uncommonly, other signs are present: diminution of vibration and position sense, unsteadiness, poor muscular coordination with ataxia, moodiness, mental slowness, poor memory, confusion, agitation and depression, delusions, hallucinations, psychosis (usually with paranoid ideation) and central scotomata, sometimes with dim vision due to optic atrophy or tobacco amblyopia.[13, 33, 439, 444–446, 446a] The wide variety of sensory and motor changes tend to be symmetric, especially if maintained for a period of weeks or months.[447] This is not invariably so, however.

In the author's experience, loss of position sense in the index toes, and loss of vibration sense, as tested by a 256 vibrations per second tuning fork, usually precedes by many months any evidence of loss of position sense in the great toes or of vibration sense with a 128 vibrations per second tuning fork. Recently, a patient with addisonian pernicious anemia in relapse was seen who had just been given a clean bill of health by an excellent neurologist. Examination with a "256" tuning fork revealed complete loss of vibration sense from toes to iliac crests bilaterally, although the neurologist's finding of "no loss of vibration sense" (using a "128" tuning fork) was confirmed. Also, while the neurologist's finding of "no loss of position sense" (in the great toes) was confirmed, position sense was absent in both index toes. The author has not been able to find in the literature the incidence of loss of "256" vibration sense and index toe position sense in a random sampling of the population, and so cannot state with certainty that these findings by themselves are of great significance. They do seem to have a definite relation to early vitamin B_{12} deficiency disease, and, when present with such deficiency, usually disappear after treatment with vitamin B_{12}.

It is extremely important to realize that nervous system involvement may occur in the absence of overt anemia. Such involvement may be present for years and irreversible damage may occur if the proper diagnosis is made too late.[33, 444-449]

In the author's experience with cases of vitamin B_{12} deficiency disease with neurologic involvement in the absence of overt anemia (and of folic acid administration), careful examination of the peripheral blood always revealed the presence of an increase over the normal number of neutrophilic polymorpho-nuclear leukocytes with hypersegmented nuclei, and also some macroovalocytosis (see CHAPTER 3). Examination of the bone marrow revealed changes suggesting early megaloblastic hemato-poiesis: large erythrocyte precursors with less than the usual amount of clumping of the nuclear chromatin, especially in the early stages of development (i.e., intermediate megaloblasts), and large but perhaps not quite giant metamyelocytes.

Information as to the existence of similar hematologic clues in the reported cases of vitamin B_{12} deficiency with nervous system involvement and no overt anemia is sparse. It is quite possible that similar findings were present, but not commented upon, as was the case in one report.[449]

The importance of these hematologic clues is best illustrated by case reports:

F. McL., a 63 year old white man of Irish parentage, was first seen at the Monte-fiore Hospital in May, 1958, when he was admitted to the semiprivate service for evaluation of a recent progression of Parkinson's disease, which had been only slowly progressive during the past five years. He lived alone, ate a poor diet, drank a quart of beer daily, and had at one time been an alcoholic. For three years he had manifested steadily progressive mental confusion and forgetfulness. On several occasions he had wandered out into the street and not known where he was. At times he had gone to work on holidays when his place of work was closed. His judgment was noted by relatives to be progressively poorer.

On admission he was obese and plethoric, and mildly confused and disoriented. Slight hepatomegaly was noted. Routine examination of the peripheral blood revealed a hematocrit of 41.5 per cent, hemoglobin 13.8 Gm., red cell count (obtained after examination of the peripheral blood smear suggested the proper diagnosis) 3.1 million, white cell count 4,700, with 58 per cent neutrophilic polymorphonuclear leukocytes, 24 per cent lymphocytes, 8 per cent monocytes, and 10 per cent eosinophils. Marked macroovalocytosis and a slight increase in the number of neutrophilic polymorphonuclear leukocytes with hypersegmented nuclei were noted.

Because of the peripheral blood findings, a sternal bone marrow aspirate was obtained. Some large, but no giant, metamyelocytes were seen; some of the erythroid precursors were large with nuclear chromatin more finely divided than that normally seen. Not one of the 10 hematologists to whom the specimen was submitted for examination believed that the marrow could be classified as megaloblastic. Indeed, one hematologist of wide experience who examined the specimens, after being asked to look at them for evidences of vitamin B_{12} deficiency, stated: "There is a mild erythroid hyperplasia without maturation arrest; this specimen is not consistent with vitamin B_{12} deficiency."

Nonetheless, serum was obtained for assay of vitamin B_{12} content, and a urinary excretion test of a modified Schilling type was started.[450, 451] Prior to and shortly after the start of this test, the patient dressed and attempted to leave the hospital without notifying anyone. On the first occasion he was brought back to his ward by a police officer who found him wandering aimlessly on the street. The patient claimed he left because there were "thirty people after him." A psychiatrist called in consultation made the diagnosis of an "organic psychosis associated with cerebral arteriosclerosis."

Because of the necessity for constant supervision, and despite the fact that a definite lessening of his confusion was noticeable within two days after the first 1 mg. injection of vitamin B_{12}, given in the course of the urinary vitamin B_{12} excretion test, it was considered necessary that he be transferred to a mental institution. Transfer was arranged to the closed psychiatric ward of the Bronx Municipal Hospital Center.

At this time the study results were obtained. The serum B_{12} level was 96 $\mu\mu$g./ml. by Euglena gracilis assay.[452] This low result was coupled with the result of the urinary excretion test and the diagnosis of pernicious anemia was made. (The urinary excretion test demonstrated that the patient lacked intrinsic factor, since he excreted only 0.76 per cent of the orally administered dose of labeled vitamin B_{12} when it was given alone, but 10.2 per cent of the dose when it was given with a standard amount of hog intrinsic factor concentrate.)

These results were communicated to the staff of the closed psychiatric ward where the patient resided, and treatment was instituted with 1 mg. of vitamin B_{12} daily. After three weeks of such treatment, his psychiatric status had improved to the point that it was feasible to discharge him with the diagnosis of "incipient addisonian pernicious anemia with cerebral vitamin B_{12} deficiency, improved by treatment."

Had the significance of the macroovalocytes and hyperseg- mented polymorphonuclear leukocytes in the peripheral blood of this patient been overlooked, he would have probably spent the rest of his life in a mental institution as "just another case of senile psychosis."

Part of this patient's mental disturbance may have been re- lated to factors other than vitamin B_{12} deficiency, since he had been a chronic alcoholic and since the possibility of some cere- bral arteriosclerosis did exist. It is always difficult to be certain that a psychosis or other neurologic system damage derived purely from vitamin B_{12} deficiency. The major criterion is response to vitamin B_{12} therapy. Unless such response is com- plete, it may be impossible to determine how much of the failure to return to complete normality is due to irreversible damage related to the length of time the patient was deficient in vitamin B_{12} and how much is due to other causes. This problem fre- quently arises in the many patients with both pernicious anemia and diabetes mellitus, either of which is capable of producing severe peripheral neuropathy.

Another case in which vitamin B_{12} deficiency appeared almost certainly to be the only agent involved in the psychosis now follows:

The patient was a 39 year old man who was seen by a psychiatrist in March, 1957 because of slight ataxia and paranoid ideation. Diminished position and vibration sense in the lower extremities were noted, but not further evaluated in terms of possible vitamin B_{12} deficiency. The patient became increasingly paranoid, and in September, 1957 was admitted to a private sanitarium for treat- ment of "paranoid schizophrenia" which was clearly evident even to the casual observer. One day, in December, 1957, after he had received 17 electroshock treatments with "mild benefit," it was noted that he was pale. Hematologic workup revealed a megaloblastic anemia with a hemoglobin of 5.8 Gm./100 ml. of blood. He was started on treatment with vitamin B_{12} and transferred to the Bronx Municipal Hospital Center, from which institution he was discharged in seven weeks no longer psychotic or anemic, with a proved diagnosis of addisonian pernicious anemia, to return to his wife and children.

Had he not been lucky enough to develop an anemia severe enough to be recognized with the unaided eye, this man might have gone on to develop irreversible cerebral damage, as well as severe combined-system disease.

These cases, and many others seen by the author and many prior workers, emphasize the importance of screening psychotic patients for vitamin B_{12} deficiency by careful examination of the peripheral blood smear, determination of the serum vitamin B_{12} level, or both.[33, 446a] Such a screening procedure, carried out at large mental institutions, might prove of sufficient value to pay for itself many times over in saved patient-days. Similar screening might prove fruitful in patients whose mental changes are not serious enough to require hospitalization, but in whom "senility" is considered to explain adequately their behavior.

Another case demonstrating the importance of careful examination of the peripheral blood smear as a routine procedure, while perhaps not as dramatic as the first case, now follows:

M. L., a 45 year old lady, was admitted to the semiprivate service of the Montefiore Hospital in April, 1958 for evaluation because of an attack of syncope. Similar episodes of syncope had occurred intermittently for the three years prior to admission, and there had been a single syncopal episode 20 years previously.

Routine hematologic workup revealed a hematocrit of 33.5 per cent, hemoglobin 12.4 Gm., red count 3.35 million, and white count 4,400 with 60 per cent neutrophilic polymorphonuclear leukocytes, 32 per cent lymphocytes, 4 per cent eosinophils, and 4 per cent monocytes. Marked anisocytosis was noted, with macroovalocytes and a slight increase in the number of neutrophilic polymorphonuclear leukocytes with hypersegmented nuclei. An occasional Howell-Jolly body was seen.

Because of these findings a sternal bone marrow aspirate was obtained. This showed "an occasional overly large metamyelocyte and some lagging of maturation of the nucleus in some of the red cell precursors; also a moderate eosinophilia."

Unfortunately, vitamin B_{12} administration was begun immediately on notification of the suspected diagnosis, and serum was not obtained for vitamin B_{12} assay. However, urinary excretion testing [450] revealed that only 1.13 per cent of an oral, labeled dose of vitamin B_{12} was excreted; this was raised to 11.07 per cent when the oral vitamin B_{12} dose was supplemented with hog intrinsic factor concentrate.

The diagnosis of early addisonian pernicious anemia was made and the patient was discharged on maintenance injections of vitamin B_{12}.

It is of interest that the diagnosis could have been made two years earlier. In 1956 the patient had a single episode of Henoch-Schonlein purpura, with melena and microscopic hematuria. She was hospitalized throughout the course of that episode. Seven hematocrits ranged from 32 to 36 per cent, and reticulocyte counts varied from 0.7 to 2.2 per cent. No red counts or hemoglobin determinations were made. A bone marrow aspirate was obtained and reported as showing "myeloid hyperplasia with eosinophilia," and nothing else of interest. However, review of that marrow specimen at Montefiore Hospital in 1958 revealed the presence of large metamyelocytes and red cell precursors with more finely divided chromatin than normal (i.e., intermediate megaloblasts), such as were seen in the bone marrow aspirated in 1958.

Of further interest is the fact that, when an episode of syncope occurred during the 1956 hospitalization, a thorough neurologic examination was performed. The findings were: "Vibration slightly depressed at ankles. Ankle jerks absent. Hypoaesthesia distal phalanx, left middle finger. May have mild peripheral neuropathy, evidence equivocal."

Had the hematologic and neurologic findings been given the attention they deserved, the diagnosis of addisonian pernicious anemia would have been made two years earlier. Luckily, in this particular instance there was no marked progression of the neurologic damage during the period of delay, and no permanent irreversible damage was done. Incidentally, hypersegmented polymorphonuclear leukocytes and macrocytes were noted in the 1956 bone marrow specimen when it was reviewed two years later, and they were undoubtedly also present in the peripheral blood. In only one of the six peripheral blood smear reports obtained in 1956 was the presence of macrocytes noted (and ignored); the presence of hypersegmented polymorphonuclear leukocytes was not even mentioned.

The most prominent symptoms and signs of vitamin B_{12} deficiency disease are recorded in TABLES 3 AND 4, adapted from

TABLE 3.—*Symptoms of Vitamin B_{12} Deficiency Disease*

| | Pre-Liver Series | | Edinburgh Series 1944–56 Davidson |
	1908 Cabot, Boston	1923 Panton, London	
No. of cases	1,200	117	250
Weakness and tiredness	96%	91%	90%
Dyspnoea	88%	—	70%
Sore tongue	43% (of 372 cases)	24% (of 34 cases)	25%
Diarrhoea	51%	26%	9%
Constipation	35%	—	16%
Paraesthesiae	100%	—	38%

TABLE 4.—*Signs of Vitamin B_{12} Deficiency Disease*

| | Pre-Liver Series | | Edinburgh Series 1944–56 Davidson |
	1908 Cabot, Boston	1923 Panton, London	
No. of cases	1,200	117	250
Fever	79%	71%	22%
"Icterus"	Most cases	—	Uncommon
Acute glossitis (red and ulcerated)	42% (of 372 cases)	—	5%
Chronic atrophic glossitis (pale and smooth)	—	—	64%
Splenomegaly	27%	18%	8%
Spinal cord damage	11%	—	7%
Asiatic type	7%	—	6%
Spastic type	4%	—	1%
Peripheral blood:			
<2 million R.B.C./c.mm.	86%	Average 1.39 million	58%
<1 million R.B.C./c.mm.	21%		1%

From DAVIDSON, S.: Clinical picture of pernicious anaemia prior to introduction of liver therapy in 1926 and in Edinburgh subsequent to 1944. Brit. M. J. *1*:241, 1957.

Sir Stanley Davidson's recent article on the differences in the clinical picture of pernicious anemia before and since the introduction of liver therapy.[439] These differences are due to generally earlier diagnosis in those geographic areas where adequate facilities for such early diagnosis exist. In those areas where such facilities either do not exist or are not used to advantage, the frequency of the various signs and symptoms of vitamin B_{12} deficiency approximates that observed in the preliver era.

The most frequent initial symptoms are weakness, dyspnea, paresthesia, and sore tongue, any or all of which may precede the onset of overt anemia by years.

An 82 year old woman had wandered from clinic to clinic for 12 years complaining of constant tingling in her hands, weakness, and occasionally a sore tongue and dyspnea. Infrequent hemoglobin determinations were always above 10 Gm./100 ml. of blood. The usual diagnosis made was "neurosis," and multivitamins (sometimes containing folic acid) were the usual therapy. When finally seen at the Bronx Municipal Hospital Center, she had gross generalized neurologic damage and marked megaloblastic anemia with a hemoglobin of 4.6 Gm. She stated her skin color had been lemon-yellow for at least two years. The diagnosis of vitamin B_{12} deficiency disease was made, and confirmed by a serum vitamin B_{12} level of 70 $\mu\mu g./ml.$ (L. Leishmanii assay).[372, 453] Failure to absorb vitamin B_{12} was demonstrated by a modified Schilling test,[459] but it was not possible subsequently to determine whether the absorptive defect was correctible by exogenous intrinsic factor because the patient developed vomiting and diarrhea, and died in uremia associated with a chronic pyelonephritis after a period of rising BUN and impaired consciousness.

When this case was being prepared for presentation at a clinical-pathologic conference, the records of the various clinics in which she had been seen during the preceding 12 years were examined. Each of the many times she was seen by a new doctor, comment was recorded of her complaints of paresthesia, weakness, and dyspnea. Not once was vitamin B_{12} deficiency considered. Yet, persistent symmetrical paresthesias of the fingers (or toes) are a major clue to the possible existence of vitamin B_{12} deficiency, and thorough evaluation of this possibility is always indicated.[443]

The folic acid deficiency states present a similar clinical picture to that of vitamin B_{12} deficiency, with the exceptions noted at the beginning of this chapter. "Pure" folic acid deficiency is rarely seen, and the actual clinical picture usually observed is that of folic acid deficiency combined with other deficiencies, and often associated with gross disorder of gastrointestinal function.

In the malabsorption syndrome, the most frequent symptoms are diarrhea, weakness, and weight loss, all of which occur in more than 4 of every 5 patients.[454] Glossitis occurs in approximately half the cases, paresthesia in almost 20 per cent, and mental symptoms in about 10 per cent. The neurologic symptoms are possibly due in large part if not completely to associated vitamin B_{12} deficiency.

The major symptoms and signs of the malabsorption syndrome are noted in TABLE 5 AND 6, adapted from a presenta-

TABLE 5.—*Major Symptoms of the Malabsorption Syndrome*

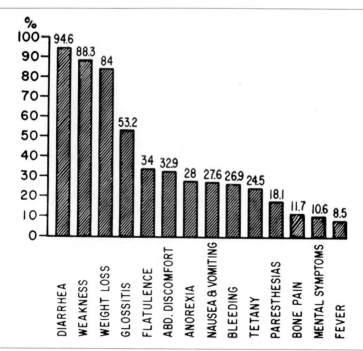

From BOSSAK, E. T., WANG, C. I., AND ADLERSBERG, D.: Clinical aspects of the malabsorption syndrome (idiopathic sprue). J. Mount Sinai Hosp. (New York) 24:286, 1957. Simultaneously published in ADLERSBERG, D., ED.: The Malabsorption Syndrome. New York, Grune and Stratton, 1957.

TABLE 6.—*Major Signs of the Malabsorption Syndrome*

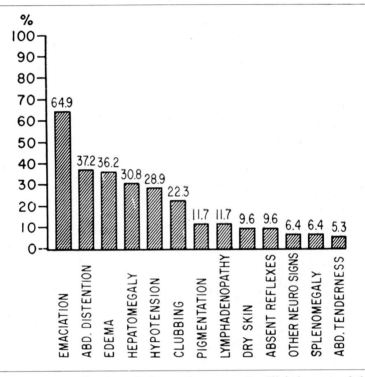

From Bossak, E. T., Wang, C. I., and Adlersberg, D.: Clinical aspects of the malabsorption syndrome (idiopathic sprue). J. Mount Sinai Hosp. (New York) *24*:286, 1957. Simultaneously published in Adlersberg, D., Ed.: The Malabsorption Syndrome. New York, Grune and Stratton, 1957.

tion[454] at a recent symposium on the malabsorption syndrome held at the Mount Sinai Hospital, New York.

The clinical picture in those conditions, other than the vitamin B_{12} or folic acid deficiency states, which are sometimes associated with a megaloblastic marrow, is that of the underlying condition (hemolytic anemia, etc.).

Pernicious anemia is associated with an increased incidence of carcinoma of the stomach, as noted in the section, "Lesions which Destroy the Gastric Mucosa," and this entity must be looked for in every patient with addisonian pernicious anemia. It is also of importance that every patient with cancer of the stomach be evaluated for possible vitamin B_{12} deficiency caused by inability to produce intrinsic factor.

The incidence of gall bladder disease in patients with pernicious anemia is considerably greater than chance.[455-457] This may be due in large part to the fact that pernicious anemia is a hemolytic anemia, in addition to being an anemia with inadequate production of circulating erythrocytes.[24, 458] In pernicious anemia there is an increased random destruction of not only the patient's own erythrocytes, but also of transfused normal red cells.[459] The resulting hyperbilirubinemia leads to an increased concentration of bilirubin in the bile, with a large amount of bile pigment from sources other than the mature circulating erythrocytes,[460] perhaps arising mainly from rapidly destroyed young erythrocytes.[460a] This in turn may lead to the precipitation of pigment in the gall bladder, cholelithiasis, and cholecystitis.[461, 461a]

The serum bilirubin of untreated patients with addisonian pernicious anemia is generally in the range of 1 mg./100 ml.,[462] and may or may not be of a degree sufficient to produce the light lemon yellow skin coloration classically associated with untreated pernicious anemia.

Clear-cut relationships between pernicious anemia per se and diseases other than those already mentioned have not yet been established but may exist. One such disease is gouty arthritis.[462a] It is obvious, however, that the fortuitous presence of another disease can alter the usual clinical picture of any of the megaloblastic anemias.

Acute liver destruction, such as occurs with acute hepatitis, may completely mask vitamin B_{12} deficiency disease.[463, 464] The liver damage releases residual vitamin B_{12} stores into the blood stream,[465] and apparently thereby makes them available for hematopoiesis.

7 *Differential Diagnosis*

I. CLINICAL

THE SINGLE MOST USEFUL TOOL in separating the megaloblastic anemias is an adequate history. This should include detailed inquiry into the quantity of animal protein and fresh green vegetables consumed in an average week. The author has seen the comment, "diet adequate," on the charts of 3 patients with megaloblastic anemia of "obscure etiology." Conversation with the patients revealed that 2 of them had substituted alcohol for almost all solid food for periods in excess of a year, and the third was a strict vegetarian! The first 2 had dietary folic acid deficiency associated with chronic alcoholism and cirrhosis; the third had dietary vitamin B_{12} deficiency. The proper diagnosis was confirmed by appropriate tests and response to therapy in all 3 patients.

Familiarity with the most frequent causes of megaloblastic anemia in various geographic areas helps in differential diagnosis. Every physician should be familiar with the most common causes of megaloblastic anemia in his own area. For example, in the New York metropolitan area, the two most common causes of megaloblastic anemia are pernicious anemia and the malabsorption syndrome, in their various subdivisions (see CHAPTER 4). The malabsorption syndrome is the most common cause of megaloblastic anemia in that large segment of the New York City population composed of recent migrants from Puerto Rico; pernicious anemia is more common in the rest of the New York population generally.

Age is important: pernicious anemia is very uncommon under the age of 40 (see CHAPTER 1).[14] Origin of the patient should be ascertained: persons from the Scandinavian countries are more likely to have pernicious anemia or fish tapeworm anemia; those from England, Ireland, and Canada have a greater chance of having pernicious anemia; patients from India may have nutritional vitamin B_{12} deficiency because of religious dietary restrictions (those with nutritional folic acid deficiency due to dietary inadequacy because of poverty are less likely to travel).

The presence of nervous system involvement indicates vitamin B_{12} deficiency. Nervous system damage due solely to folic acid deficiency, with concomitant vitamin B_{12} deficiency adequately excluded, has never been described in the literature, to the author's knowledge, and the author has never seen such a case. In the presence of a megaloblastic anemia, barring the fortuitous presence of unrelated neurologic disease, nervous system involvement indicates vitamin B_{12} deficiency with or without concomitant folic acid deficiency. It never indicates folic acid deficiency alone. This delineation is so clear that it has been suggested that neurologic damage associated with megaloblastic anemia be referred to as "vitamin B_{12} neuropathy." [420]

Each of the symptoms and signs of nervous system involvement mentioned in CHAPTER 5 should be looked for carefully, since only one or two may be present. This is especially true in vitamin B_{12} deficiency without overt megaloblastic anemia, when only careful examination of the peripheral blood smear suggests the diagnosis.

If the patient has been taking multivitamins containing folic acid, especially if the amount of folic acid in them is in excess of 0.50 mg. per day, the peripheral blood picture may be almost or even completely normal. It is quite possible that the lack of parallelism between the degree of hematopoietic and nervous system damage in vitamin B_{12} deficiency states is primarily a function of the highly variable dietary folic acid ingestion (and possibly absorption as well) from patient to patient. Regardless of diet, however, the author has never seen a patient with vitamin B_{12} neuropathy, not taking multivitamins, who did not have macroovalocytes and hypersegmented polymorphonuclear leukocytes in the peripheral blood.

Diarrhea strongly suggests the malabsorption syndrome and folic acid deficiency, often accompanied by vitamin B_{12} deficiency. However, it should be remembered that diarrhea also occurs not infrequently in pernicious anemia.[443] Conversely, the absence of diarrhea rules against the malabsorption syndrome, but does not exclude it.[465a]

This is especially true of adult coeliac disease, of which many cases have been described with bowel movements appearing normal in both quality and quantity.[384, 454, 466, 467] Some of these cases had macrocytosis; in a few a megaloblastic marrow was described. The author has seen 2 patients with megaloblastic anemia related to occult adult coeliac disease. Both had single daily normal formed stools, no history of diarrhea, low serum vitamin B_{12} and "folic acid" levels, intrinsic factor in their gastric juice by in vitro "assay," and inability to absorb an oral test dose of radioactive vitamin B_{12} either without or with added hog intrinsic factor concentrate. In both, balance studies revealed defective fat absorption and produced steatorrhea. In both patients, the megaloblastic anemia disappeared after intramuscular vitamin B_{12} administration and oral folic acid therapy. Similar cases, including one with only partial remission after combined vitamin B_{12} and folic acid administration, were reported prior to the wide availability of serum vitamin B_{12} determinations and description of the Schilling test.[384]

In pregnant women and infants, folic acid deficiency is by far the most likely cause of megaloblastic anemia.

When the usual signs and symptoms of vitamin B_{12} or folic acid deficiency are lacking, more obscure causes of megaloblastic-like anemia must be sought. These include hidden malignancies, especially leukemia, and hemolytic anemias of various types.

Thorough knowledge of the information contained in CHAPTERS 4 and 5 will make differential diagnosis of the megaloblastic anemias a relatively simple matter for the careful clinician. In areas where laboratory confirmation of the diagnosis is unavailable, therapeutic trial constitutes the time-honored method of differentiating the folic acid deficiency states from those due to vitamin B_{12} deficiency.[444]

Therapeutic trial carries with it the danger that either vitamin B_{12} or folic acid may produce a temporary remission in patients whose primary deficiency is of the other agent, thus leading the physician into improper therapy (see CHAPTER 8). For this reason, only a single small dose, or single small daily doses, should be given to the patient in such a trial.

The patient should be maintained on a diet low in folic acid and vitamin B_{12} for at least two days prior to the test (preferably for a week), and throughout the test period. A single 1 μg. injection of vitamin B_{12} is then given, and the reticulocyte count observed daily or at least every other day for seven to 12 days.[468] If there is no reticulocytosis of significance, the patient is next given 0.5 mg. of folic acid subcutaneously and reticulocytosis sought as previously.

Daily doses of 0.4 mg. of folic acid for 10 days have proved acceptable in therapeutic trials. Such a course of therapy induces hematologic response only in patients with folic acid deficiency.[468a] More study of the relative value of a single small dose of vitamin B_{12} or folic acid vs. daily small doses in therapeutic trials is needed. Daily small doses may be more reliable.

Variants of the procedure, using similar oral rather than parenteral small doses of each vitamin, may be used to test absorption, provided the status of the patient is good enough to allow the time to carry out peroral studies of about one week each prior to parenteral vitamin administration. (Peroral studies should be performed first because parenteral administration of the appropriate vitamin will always produce a greater reticulocyte response, and the method of "serial reticulocyte responses" to test agents should be carried out with the weaker agent given first. One μg of vitamin B_{12} given by mouth is less potent than the same dose parenterally because even in a completely normal subject complete absorption from the gastrointestinal tract is rare; the same is true of oral versus parenteral doses of folic acid.)

II. LABORATORY [468b]

A. Gastric Acidity

The most widely used laboratory aid to the separation of the megaloblastic anemias is the determination of gastric acidity.[469]

If the patient is over the age of 50, the presence of free acid almost rules out pernicious anemia completely; if he is under 50, then the presence of free acid makes pernicious anemia less likely, but does not rule it out entirely.[131-133]

Achlorhydria in a patient past the age of 40 is of only moderate significance in terms of the possibility of pernicious anemia. Approximately 15 per cent of people between the ages of 40 and 60 have histamine-refractory achlorhydria, as do about 25 per cent of individuals between ages 60 and 70 and 30 per cent of persons over the age of 70.[470]

Since intubation of the patient is unpleasant, tubeless gastric analysis has become popular.[471, 472] While this method for determination of gastric acidity is simple, it is unreliable in the presence of renal disease, gastric obstruction, diarrhea, and malabsorption syndrome,[473] as well as in gastrectomized patients and individuals with a rapid gastric emptying time.

Tubeless gastric analysis involves the ingestion by the patient of a cation exchange resin to which is bound quininium, azure A, or another cation. If there is free acid in the stomach, the hydrogen ions will replace the cation on the resin, which will then be absorbed into the blood stream and released in the urine, where its quantity may be measured and thereby provide a measure of the amount of hydrogen ions (i.e., of free acid) in the stomach. Unfortunately, cations in the small intestine will also exchange with the cation on the resin, making it important to examine only the urine voided within two hours of ingestion of the resin, which will contain only cation which was released in the stomach. However, if the patient has a fast gastric emptying time, even the urine voided within two hours of ingestion of the resin may contain cation released in the small intestine, and an erroneous impression of free acid in the stomach may be given.

Unexplained results "positive for free acid" have occurred in the presence of achlorhydria proven by intubation frequently enough to make the azure A resin test of dubious value in the detection of diseases associated with achlorhydria.[474] The author has seen 2 patients with pernicious anemia in whom the correct diagnosis was "ruled out" by an intelligent house staff because the presence of free acid was reported on tubeless gastric analysis with azure A resin. The diagnosis was "ruled back in" by insisting on intubation, and demonstrating the absence of free acid in the gastric aspirate. It is unknown whether the erroneous results were due to an error in technic, such as chewing of the resin granules by the patients or collection of the urine specimen more than two hours after ingestion of the resin.

Although tubeless gastric analysis using azure A resin cannot at present be recommended, the older tubeless method, using a quininium resin, appears to be more reliable, and may be a useful screening procedure.[471, 474]

B. Assay of Intrinsic Factor in Gastric Juice

In vivo assay of intrinsic factor content of gastric juice is accomplished by taking the gastric aspirate from a donor (the patient) and giving it to a recipient who is known to have no intrinsic factor, along with a small dose of radioactive vitamin B_{12}, in a Schilling type test (see G below). Alternatively, the donor's gastric juice may be given to an untreated patient with known pernicious anemia, along with 1 $\mu g.$ of vitamin B_{12}. A hematologic response of the recipient, unless due to a fortuitous spontaneous remission, would rule out lack of intrinsic factor in the donor.

In vitro "assay" of intrinsic factor in human gastric juice has been reported recently.[475, 476] This procedure obviates the need for more than a few ml. of gastric juice from the patient, and also eliminates the need for a recipient. In the author's hands, when the gastric juice has been frozen immediately after collection, this "assay" has proved generally accurate as an indication of the presence or absence of intrinsic factor in the gastric juice of achlorhydric patients. Great care in interpretation of results is required, especially in the presence of mucus (including salivary mucus), which binds vitamin B_{12},[477, 478] or of bile, which may contain nonradioactive vitamin B_{12}.[479, 480] Free acid and pepsin release nonradioactive vitamin B_{12} from the liver, thereby producing false low results. The "assay" using liver homogenate,[476] rather than liver slices,[475] has proven especially susceptible to errors introduced by these various factors, and cannot at present be recommended. Other sources of error in both "assays" include the variable amount of vitamin B_{12} in gastric juice (from less than 40 $\mu\mu$g./ml. to more than 1500 $\mu\mu$g./ml. in our laboratory), and the variable amount of what may be degraded intrinsic factor in the gastric juice. This latter material appears able to block the receptors for intrinsic factor on liver, but it appears unable to then bind vitamin B_{12}.[173a]

Evaluation in other laboratories will indicate any general usefulness of the in vitro procedure. So far, it seems to be specific for intrinsic factor. In vitro assay procedures for intrinsic factor must be evaluated very cautiously. The first such procedure [481] proved to be nonspecific,[564] and to measure only vitamin B_{12} binding,[206] a property common to many substances. That procedure conveyed the erroneous impression that intrinsic factor is lacking in patients with sprue to an even greater extent than in patients with pernicious anemia.[482] In point of fact, only those patients with sprue who also have gastric atrophy have a lack of intrinsic factor as a significant etiologic factor in their megaloblastic anemia.[3] Numerous observers have demonstrated intrinsic factor to be present usually in the gastric juice of patients with malabsorption syndrome by in vivo assay.[115, 158, 173, 245]

C. Vitamin B_{12} Serum Levels

Microbiologic assay of serum vitamin B_{12} concentration is rather widely available in large medical centers, but not yet elsewhere. The procedure is extremely useful as an objective estimate of the degree of vitamin B_{12} deficiency.[372, 453]

A number of different assay microorganisms, with varying degrees of specificity for vitamin B_{12}, have been used to determine serum vitamin B_{12} concentrations.[70, 264, 452, 453, 483-485] Results vary in different laboratories, but are generally reproducible in any one laboratory (see TABLES 7 AND 8). Determination of whether a given result represents a low serum vitamin B_{12} level should be based on normal controls in the same laboratory, not on results in other laboratories.

Ochromonas malhamensis is the most specific assay organism. Euglena gracilis is next in specificity, first in sensitivity. Lactobacillus leishmanii and Escherichia coli are less specific and sen-

TABLE 7.—*Serum Vitamin B_{12} Concentrations in Normal Subjects*

Author	Date	Number of subjects	Serum B_{12} ($\mu\mu$g./ml.)		Test organism
			Range	Mean	
Ross	1950	12	350 to 750	490	Euglena
Mollin and Ross....	1952,4	126	100 to 900	360	Euglena
Heinrich and Lahann	1953,4	—	62 to 460	238	Euglena
Killander	1953	56	100 to 720	360	Euglena
Lear et al.	1954	20	292 to 856	532	Euglena
Pitney and Beard...	1954	57	86 to 460	212	Euglena
Rosenthal and Sarett	1952	24	80 to 420	200	L. leichmannii
Girdwood	1954	50	50 to 870	320	L. leichmannii
Nieweg et al.	1954	36	310 to 1050	—	L. leichmannii
Okuda et al.	1954	30	—	158	L. leichmannii
Unglaub et al.	1954	—	70 to 420	210	L. leichmannii
Boger et al.	1955	528	70 to 1060	560	L. leichmannii
Spray	1955	111	150 to 860	437	L. leichmannii
Grossowicz et al.	1954	30	200 to 1000	—	E. coli

Taken from MOLLIN, D. L., AND ROSS, G. I. M. (see TABLE 8, page 84).

sitive, but have the advantage of rapid growth. They provide assay results in a day as compared to a week for Ochromonas and Euglena.

The more specific organisms are generally preferable. Occasionally, a less specific organism will grow on factors other than vitamin B_{12} contained in the serum of a vitamin B_{12}-deficient patient, thereby conveying the erroneous impression that the patient is not deficient in the vitamin. We[512] have seen a patient with proved vitamin B_{12} deficiency (cerebral and hematologic involvement; classic Schilling test result) whose serum vitamin B_{12} level was only 20 $\mu\mu$g./ml. by E. gracilis assay, yet with a serum vitamin B_{12} level of 1500 $\mu\mu$g./ml. by L. leishmanii assay. The result was thrice repeated prior to treatment of the patient. A similar case has been observed by Lowenstein.[485a]

The value of determining "free B_{12}" as well as "total B_{12}" has not been established. "Free B_{12}" is that quantity of the vitamin in human serum which is available to the assay microorganism

TABLE 8.—*Serum Vitamin B_{12} Concentrations in Pernicious Anemia in Relapse*

Author	Date	Number of patients	Serum B_{12} ($\mu\mu$g./ml.)		Test organism
			Range	Mean	
Mollin and Ross....	1952,4	190	$<$16 to 105	40	Euglena
Heinrich and Lahann	1953,4	—	0.01 to 30	5	Euglena
Killander	1953	12	$<$25 to 105	38	Euglena
Lear et al.	1954	33	0 to 85	39	Euglena
Pitney and Beard...	1955	17	0 to 46	13	Euglena
Girdwood	1954	36	$<$50 to 200	95 (25) $<$50 (11)	L. leichmannii
Nieweg et al.	1954	17	$<$ 5 to 175	—	L. leichmannii
Unglaub et al.	1954	10	10 to 70	40	L. leichmannii
Spray	1955	17	? to 140	—	L. leichmannii
Grossowicz et al.	1954	8	50 — 130	75	E. coli

From MOLLIN, D. L., AND ROSS, G. I. M.: The pathophysiology of vitamin B_{12} deficiency in the megaloblastic anaemias. *In* Heinrich, H. C.: Vitamin B_{12} und Intrinsic Factor. Stuttgart, Ferdinand Enke, 1957.

prior to the routine heating of the serum to release B_{12} from serum protein. The amount of "free B_{12}" in a given sample of serum is different for different microorganisms and different durations of incubation. The physiologic significance in man of "free B_{12}" is unknown, although it is generally believed that it represents vitamin B_{12} not bound to protein or to any other substance.

Recent evidence [486, 487] indicates that in the normal individual the serum and red blood cell vitamin B_{12} levels are roughly equal. As vitamin B_{12} deficiency develops, the serum vitamin B_{12}

level falls first, and is slowly followed by the red cell vitamin B_{12} level. Thus, in 5 patients whose serum vitamin B_{12} levels had fallen to an average of 35 $\mu\mu$g./ml., the vitamin B_{12} content of the unwashed red cells still averaged 140 $\mu\mu$g./ml.[487] Further studies are needed to define the possible usefulness of determining red cell vitamin B_{12} levels as a measure of general tissue depletion of the vitamin. In such studies it must be kept in mind that "red cell" vitamin B_{12} levels may include a large fraction of vitamin B_{12} contained in leukocytes.

In early vitamin B_{12} deficiency, prior to the development of anemia and a clearly megaloblastic bone marrow, and after the appearance of macroovalocytes and an increase in number of hypersegmented neutrophilic polymorphonuclear leukocytes in the peripheral blood, serum vitamin B_{12} levels frequently have not fallen below the range of normal, although they are always well below the mean normal value.[488]

D. "Folic Acid" Serum Levels

Microbiologic assay of blood "folic acid" has fallen into disrepute since the demonstration that such assay does not measure folic acid, but rather measures a multiplicity of factors, all of which have folic acid-like activity for microorganisms, but none of which is folic acid.[288, 289] Although folic acid per se is not normally present in serum, it is accepted that what is measured in serum immediately after administration of folic acid orally or parenterally *is* folic acid itself. Theoretically, however, the only valid measure of folic acid depletion would be direct assay of tissue stores of this vitamin, as both folic and folinic acids.[34, 39] The next best measure would be assay of serum folic acid levels if such could be determined. Other laboratory procedures, such as the indirect methods discussed in the section, "Tests of Folic Acid Absorption, Stores, and Utilization" and the section, "Assay of Metabolic Products Found in the Urine of Folic Acid-Deficient Patients," must be interpreted with extreme caution. It must especially be kept in mind that since vitamin B_{12} deficiency results in deranged folic acid metabolism, the metabolic products of folic acid deficiency may be found in the urine of patients who have adequate ingestion and absorption of folic acid, but utilize it inadequately due to vitamin B_{12} deficiency. Failure to recognize this fact may lead to an erroneous diagnosis of primary folic acid deficiency when in fact the patient lacks only vitamin B_{12}. Similarly, injected or orally administered folic acid may rapidly disappear into the tissues of patients with vitamin B_{12} deficiency, and such rapid disappearance in these cases does not indicate a primary folic acid deficiency.[4]

Because of these problems of interpretation of indirect methods of assaying folic acid deficiency states, we [489, 489a, 489b] decided to investigate the possibility that the folic acid-like activity in human serum may in fact reflect the presence or absence of primary folic acid deficiency.

We have so far determined the serum "folic acid" levels of more than 100 patients with megaloblastic anemia, using a modified L. casei assay technic which is simple and rapid (the organism grows well within 24 hours). Low levels (below 5 mμg. of "folic acid" activity per ml. of serum) were found in those sera from patients proved to have primary folic acid deficiency by history, inadequate response to vitamin B_{12} therapy, and/or normal serum vitamin B_{12} levels, and excellent response to folic acid administration. Those sera from patients with primary vitamin B_{12} deficiency, proved by low serum vitamin B_{12} levels and excellent hematologic response to vitamin B_{12} therapy, had "folic acid" levels above 7 mμg./ml.[489] Some patients with primary deficiencies of both vitamins were uncovered; these patients proved to be ingesting grossly inadequate diets (often while pregnant) and/or to be suffering from malabsorption syndrome. All sera were obtained while the patients were fasting.

It is the author's belief that determination of the serum "folic acid" level may prove to rank with assay of the serum vitamin B_{12} level as a prime laboratory tool in evaluation of all patients with megaloblastic anemia.

E. Tests of Folic Acid Absorption, Stores, and Utilization

Measurable amounts of folic acid appear in the serum of individuals given oral doses of 1 mg. or more of the vitamin.[4, 312, 490–492]

Amounts of folic acid averaging less than 10 μg. daily are normally excreted in the urine.[493–495] When folic acid is administered orally or parenterally, urinary excretion is markedly increased.[336, 493, 495, 496]

These observations have been used to advantage in studying folic acid absorption, stores, and utilization.[4] Following the subcutaneous administration of 5 mg. of folic acid, the urinary excretion of less than 1.5 mg. in 24 hours is an indication of gross tissue depletion.[336] The converse is not necessarily true (i.e., urinary excretion of more than 1.5 mg. does not mean the patient is not desaturated), perhaps because of an obligatory excretion by the kidney.[259]

A similar indirect measure of the tissue stores of folic acid is determination of the rate of clearance of an intravenous dose of 15 μg. of folic acid per Kg. of the patient's body weight.[497] This dose appears to be completely cleared after 15 minutes in nearly all patients who are clinically deficient in folic acid, but not in normal control subjects. Of course, since this test measures the end result of a number of phenomena, rapid clearance of a test dose of folic acid can only be considered suggestive of folic acid deficiency, and not conclusive for it. This is equally true for any indirect test of folic acid stores.

After "saturation" of the tissues by administration of 15 mg. of folic acid subcutaneously for a week, Girdwood [336] has determined the urinary excretion of a 5 mg. oral dose. He found that the excretion of less than 1.5 mg. of folic acid in the subsequent 24 hour period was an indication of severe malabsorption.

While these results have been confirmed by Cox et al.,[498] other workers found sufficient overlap in urinary excretion after the test dose in "saturated" normal subjects and patients with malabsorption syndrome to make interpretation of the results difficult.[312] They proposed "saturation" of the folic acid-deficient patient with 20 to 40 mg. of folic acid for at least four weeks, followed by oral administration of a 3 mg. test dose and assay of the serum folic acid concentration one, two, and four hours later. In their studies, peak serum concentrations in normal subjects ranged from 42 to 170 μmg. of folic acid per ml. of serum. Peak values below 40 μmg. were found almost uniformly in patients with malabsorption syndrome.

Caution in interpreting any of these indirect tests of folic acid deficiency is warranted, to avoid making an erroneous diagnosis of primary folic acid deficiency when the patient actually is suffering from a primary vitamin B_{12} deficiency.[4] In severe vitamin B_{12} deficiency, the disappearance of ingested or injected folic acid appears to be as rapid as it is in folic acid deficiency.[4, 497]

F. Assay of Metabolic Products Found in the Urine of Folic Acid-Deficient Patients

Normally, histidine is metabolized to N-formimino-L-glutamic acid (FIGlu), which is degraded to glutamic acid in the presence of folic acid.[499, 500] Folic acid deficiency, either primary or secondary, results in excretion of undegraded FIGlu in the urine [501]; this metabolic defect may be made more striking by feeding l-histidine.[502]

When folic acid deficiency is very severe, high concentrations of unmetabolized FIGlu may be found in the urine.[503-514] In milder folic acid deficiency states, it may be necessary to give the patient l-histidine orally to induce FIGlu excretion in the urine.[509, 511] Thus, assay of the amount of FIGlu in the urine by microbiologic [504, 509] or enzymatic and spectrophotometric methods [506, 507] may prove to be a useful measure of folic acid deficiency.

Using microbiologic methods [504, 509] we [512] have not been able, without giving the patients oral load doses of l-histidine, to find FIGlu in the urine of some patients with megaloblastic anemias of infancy, pregnancy, poor diet, and malabsorption syndrome. In some of these cases we did not find FIGlu in the urine even after a "loading" dose of 5 Gm. of l-histidine. These patients were proved to be folic acid-deficient by presence of low serum "folic acid" levels, normal serum vitamin B_{12} levels, and excellent hematologic response to folic acid therapy after inadequate responses to vitamin B_{12} injection. Because of this, and because of the necessity for at least one and frequently more than one 24-hour urine collection (difficult to obtain from infants and incontinent adults) to study for FIGlu, we do not use FIGlu assay routinely in evaluation of patients with megaloblastic anemia at present.

Using the more precise enzymatic method, Hiatt did not observe FIGlu in the urine of a patient proved by therapeutic trial to have folic acid deficiency by Marshall, Jandl, and Castle; FIGlu did not appear after a 2 Gm. "loading" dose of l-histidine (personal communication). This result adds another case to the accumulating series of patients with proved folic acid deficiency who nonetheless do not excrete FIGlu in their urine.[509, 512]

It must be remembered that severe vitamin B_{12} deficiency, by interfering with folic acid metabolism, may induce FIGlu excretion.[513] * This may lead to a false diagnosis of primary folic acid deficiency (i.e., inadequate ingestion or absorption of folic acid), when in fact the only primary deficiency may be in the amount of vitamin B_{12} in the patient's body, and the patient may have only a secondary deficiency of folic acid (i.e., inadequate utilization of an adequate supply of folic acid, due to insufficient vitamin B_{12} for normal folic acid metabolism).

Recent studies [514, 514a] indicate that in folic acid-deficient animals, formic acid, possibly derived from tryptophane metabolism, also appears in the urine in high concentration. Assay of the concentration of this agent in urine may also prove of some use as an index of folic acid deficiency, again keeping in

---

* Patients with vitamin B_{12} deficiency and no determinable folic acid deficiency who nevertheless excreted FIGlu in their urine have been observed by Rucknagel, LaDu, Laster, Seegmiller, Daft, and Silverman; Marshall, Jandl, Castle, and Hiatt; and Herbert, Baker, Frank, Pasher, Wasserman, and Sobotka.

mind the caution that in severe vitamin B_{12} deficiency, folic acid metabolism may be disturbed.

G. Tests of Vitamin B_{12} Absorption

Absorption of vitamin B_{12} may be measured following the oral administration of physiologic (two μg. or less) doses of radio-active-cobalt-labeled vitamin.[3] This may be done by determining the amount of radioactivity in the feces (Heinle-Welch test),[515] the plasma,[516] the liver (Glass test),[517] or the urine (Schilling test).[451] The relative merits of these four methods have recently been carefully appraised.[3]

In terms of ease, speed of execution, and minimal retention of radioactivity by the patient, the clinically most useful test at the present time is measurement of the percentage of the oral dose subsequently found in the urine; this is generally known as the Schilling test after its originator.[451] Plasma radioactivity determination is simpler, but radioactive cobalt-labeled vitamin B_{12} of high enough specific activity for accurate measurement, in the conventional well-type counter, of a plasma sample is not widely available.

The author prefers a modified form [450, 518] of the Schilling test, because the original test requires a longer waiting period between test doses, and a two hour delay between oral and parenteral doses of vitamin B_{12}, which reduces the adaptability of the test for outpatients.[245, 519] Additionally, a single 24 hour urine collection following a single intramuscular injection of vitamin B_{12} as a "flushing" dose may occasionally lead to mis-diagnosis. Patients with renal disease have delayed vitamin B_{12} excretion, and the first 24 hour urine collection may be mis-leadingly low.[520, 521] The author has observed delayed excretion of radioactive vitamin B_{12} occasionally in the absence of any determinable renal disease. The most striking case in this regard was a 37 year old woman with transverse myelitis in whom neu-ropathy due to vitamin B_{12} deficiency was suspected, and in whom determination of the serum B_{12} level was valueless due to recent B_{12} therapy. She excreted 1.2 per cent of the oral dose in the first 24 hours, and 12 per cent in the second 24 hour period. Had a single 24 hour collection been made, the erroneous conclusion of inability to absorb vitamin B_{12} would have been made. (In a repeat test, this patient displayed a normal excretion pattern. The cause of the delayed excretion in the first test is unknown.)

The 2 μg. oral dose of radio-B_{12}, as originally proposed by Schilling,[451] is probably preferable to smaller doses. It appears to just saturate the physiologic intrinsic factor-dependent system for B_{12} absorption, which lesser doses do not.[518] This saturation results in more highly reproducible tests than those with smaller doses, which are affected more by small changes (such as mixture with small amounts of nonradioactive vitamin B_{12} in the stomach and small intestine).

Oral radio-B_{12} doses in excess of 2 μg. invalidate the Schilling test as a measure of the physiologic intrinsic factor-dependent mechanism of vitamin B_{12} absorption. A significant aliquot of such supraphysiologic doses (i.e., doses much greater than the amount of vitamin B_{12} in a well balanced meal) may be absorbed independently of the intrinsic factor-dependent system (see page 20).

The modified Schilling test is performed as follows[450, 518]: 2 μg. of radioactive cobalt-labeled vitamin B_{12} is given to the patient by mouth, separated from food by at least two hours. One mg. of nonradioactive vitamin B_{12} is injected intramuscularly immediately after the oral dose of labeled vitamin. All urine is collected in the ensuing 24 hour period. A second "flushing" injection of 1 mg. nonradioactive vitamin B_{12} is given to "wash" much of the remaining labeled vitamin out of the body, and again the urine is collected for 24 hours. The radioactivity in the two urine collections is determined in an appropriate radioactivity-counting apparatus, and recorded as "per cent of the oral dose."

If desired, the radioactivity may be concentrated by evaporation[522] or more difficult methods[523] prior to counting. The evaporation procedure[522] consists in thorough mixing of the entire 24 hour urine collection, measurement of the total volume, and transfer of a 500 ml. aliquot to a 1 or 2 liter Erlenmeyer flask. Twenty-five ml. of concentrated nitric acid are added to the aliquot, and it is heated to boiling with the addition of boiling chips as needed. The nitric acid appears to inactivate the components of the urine responsible for foaming, thus allowing the urine to boil vigorously on a hot plate without foaming over. Boiling is continued until the total volume is less than 50 ml., at which time it is transferred to a suitable container and made up to 50 ml. with tap water. This volume is suitable for counting on a flat scintillation crystal, the most inexpensive type available.

If the amount of radioactivity excreted in 48 hours is below the range of normal, careful inquiry is made to exclude a "false low" invalid result caused by loss of the radioactive vitamin B_{12} orally (vomiting), rectally (diarrhea), or by incomplete urine collection. A valid low result means the patient is absorbing an inadequate quantity of vitamin B_{12} because of either gastric or intestinal disorder, and repetition of the entire 48 hour procedure is mandatory, with the patient this time ingesting a standard dose of hog (or human) intrinsic factor concentrate with the oral dose of radioactive vitamin B_{12}.

This second test period allows division of patients unable to absorb vitamin B_{12} into two groups: those whose absorption of vitamin B_{12} is corrected to normal by intrinsic factor, and those whose absorption is not so corrected. The former group includes all patients with inadequate or absent secretion of intrinsic factor as the cause of their megaloblastic anemia; the latter includes those with vitamin B_{12} deficiency due to small intestinal disorder. The former group also includes some patients with fish tapeworm; in this special situation the worms may compete successfully for vitamin B_{12} with the host's intrinsic factor supply, but may not be successful when the host's intrinsic factor is aided by an exogenous supply (especially when the radioactive vitamin is bound to the exogenous intrinsic factor before it reaches the site of localization of the tapeworm).

TABLE 9.—*Range of Urinary Excretion of an Oral Dose of 2 μg. of Radioactive Vitamin B₁₂, Measured as Per Cent of the Oral Dose*

Day	Oral Treatment	Normals	Pernicious Anemia	Sprue
1	Vitamin B$_{12}$ alone	4.1–29.2	0.0– 2.7	0.1–2.2
2		0.7–20.0	0.0– 1.5	0.1–0.6
3	B$_{12}$+Intrinsic Factor	3.6–22.4	2.0–16.4	0.2–1.5
4		1.4–12.8	0.1–10.3	0.1–1.1

TABLES 9 AND 10 delineate the range and average of the urinary radioactive vitamin B$_{12}$ excretion in normal subjects, patients with pernicious anemia, and patients with malabsorption syndrome ("sprue syndrome"), as determined by Ellenbogen and Williams (personal communication) for the modification of the Schilling test described above.[450, 518] In general terms, normal 48 hour values are never below 5 per cent of the 2 μg. oral dose, and values below 3 per cent invariably indicate defective absorption. Tests giving results between 3 per cent and 5 per cent should be repeated.

As a general rule, in pernicious anemia the excretion of radioactive vitamin B$_{12}$ should be increased at least fivefold by the addition of intrinsic factor. In malabsorption syndrome, the addition of intrinsic factor may occasionally increase the excretion of vitamin B$_{12}$ as much as twofold (e.g., excretion over 48 hours may be 2 per cent with B$_{12}$ alone and 4 per cent with added intrinsic factor).

Recent work [3, 140] raises the question as to whether it is of

TABLE 10.—*Average Urinary Excretion of an Oral Dose of 2 μg. of Radioactive Vitamin B₁₂, Measured as Per Cent of the Oral Dose.*

Day	Oral Treatment	Normals	Pernicious Anemia	Sprue
1	Vitamin B$_{12}$ alone	10.5 (64)	0.7 (124)	0.7 (7)
2		4.4 (45)	0.3 (100)	0.3 (6)
3	B$_{12}$+Intrinsic Factor	12.1 (23)	7.2 (128)	0.7 (8)
4		5.3 (20)	3.3 (117)	0.4 (8)

Figures in parentheses represent the number of patients.

The author is indebted to Drs. L. Ellenbogen and W. L. Williams for TABLES 9 and 10.

clinical value to repeat the Schilling-type test a third time, using an oral dose of radioactive vitamin B_{12} and simultaneous injection of 0.25 mg. of carbamylcholine chloride (Carbachol). This third test would be reserved for those patients with inadequate secretion of intrinsic factor causing inadequate vitamin B_{12} absorption correctible by addition of intrinsic factor. Carbachol, by stimulating gastric secretion of intrinsic factor, would separate those patients *capable* of secreting an adequate quantity of intrinsic factor from those *not* capable of doing so.

Such separation is of great value in helping to understand the cloudy etiology of the varying forms of pernicious anemia (see CHAPTER 4) and is an extremely desirable research undertaking. In terms of clinical usefulness, however, such separation may not be of great value, since regardless of whether or not the patient is *capable* of secreting intrinsic factor under intensive stimulus with Carbachol, if such secretion does not occur *in physiologic circumstances* the patient will develop megaloblastic anemia due to vitamin B_{12} deficiency. This is well illustrated in a case report.[138]

For this reason, plus the fact that Carbachol is a very powerful parasympathomimetic agent which may be used only with great care in patients who are seriously ill,[548] Carbachol stimulation is not recommended for routine use in evaluation of patients with megaloblastic anemia. After the anemia has been adequately treated, providing the patient has no complicating disorder, it would be of interest to determine the effect of Carbachol on vitamin B_{12} absorption.

It must be kept in mind constantly that, while the Schilling test is used as a measure of vitamin B_{12} absorption, it in fact measures the end product of the processes of absorption, transport, retention, and renal excretion of the vitamin. Anything affecting any of these four major variables will affect the test result. Thus, before concluding that absorption of vitamin B_{12} has been measured, it must be ascertained that there are no abnormalities of the other three variables.

8 *Therapy*

PROPER TREATMENT of any of the megaloblastic anemias follows accurate differential diagnosis. Since nearly all of the megaloblastic anemias are due to deficiency of vitamin B_{12}, folic acid, or both, either or both of these agents provide specific therapy in most cases.

In the absence of complications, such as concomitant iron deficiency or another disorder affecting the hematopoietic system, adequate specific therapy is followed by a dramatically rapid hematopoietic response.[13, 25] Within a maximum period of about eight hours after the start of therapy, the megaloblasts in the bone marrow begin to be replaced by normoblasts. This process is almost complete within two days, and is nearly always complete within about a week.

In the peripheral blood, morphologic return to normal is much slower. The Arneth count "shift to the right" gradually returns to normal over a period of one or two months, and the macroovalocytes usually disappear over a period of one to three months.

The rapid generation of erythrocytes results in an outpouring of reticulocytes into the peripheral blood, with the maximal reticulocytosis being observed about the fourth to the twelfth day after the start of treatment. The larger the therapeutic dose, the earlier in this period is the maximal reticulocytosis usually observed. By the same token, the lower the patient's circulating erythrocyte count at the start of specific therapy, the greater will be the relative number of reticulocytes to mature erythrocytes in the peripheral blood (i.e., "per cent reticulocytosis") with therapy.

The rate of rise of the red cell count and the packed cell volume (hematocrit) is greatest immediately following the peak rise in the reticulocyte count. The rapidity of increase in erythrocytes then tapers off, and normal values are usually attained in approximately four to eight weeks after the start of treatment.

When circumstances allow, the hematologic response to therapy should be documented by observing the erythrocyte, leukocyte, platelet, and reticulocyte counts, the hematocrit and hemoglobin, and the appearance of the peripheral blood smear. These observations should be made just prior to the start of therapy and at weekly intervals thereafter for the first month, then every two weeks during the second month. In addition, the reticulocyte count should be determined every two days from the start of treatment until the reticulocyte peak has been passed.

Determination of the serum iron level has proved valuable in quickly assessing the effectiveness of vitamin B_{12} or folic acid therapy.[273, 524] Characteristically, the serum iron level is elevated in untreated megaloblastic anemia, regardless of whether it is due to deficiency of vitamin B_{12} or of folic acid. Within 24 hours after administration of the appropriate agent, there is nearly always an abrupt and striking fall of the serum iron; this is observed in practically all cases by 48 hours, if the therapy is adequate. Values tend to fall to about 50 to 60 μg. of iron per 100 ml. of serum within the 48 hour period, and remain at that level until the blood count returns to normal. If the therapeutic dosage is too small, the serum iron tends to rise shortly after it has fallen. If overt iron deficiency is impending, the serum iron falls to values below 40 $\mu g./100$ ml. with a range from 11 to 39 observed in 9 cases.[524]

In this connection it should be noted that the presence of a "normal" serum iron level or the presence of iron in the bone marrow of a patient with *untreated* megaloblastic anemia does not necessarily indicate adequate iron stores for maintenance of normal hematopoiesis. Generalized siderosis is frequent in megaloblastic anemia, even among peoples consuming iron-deficient diets.[409] Much of this iron may be derived from disruption of intracellular iron-containing enzymes and not from hemoglobin.[409] Therefore, only if storage iron is noted in the bone marrow *after* specific treatment of megaloblastic anemia can associated iron deficiency be ruled out.

Very slow conversion from a megaloblastic to a normoblastic marrow frequently occurs in patients with malabsorption syndrome, even when they are treated with both vitamin B_{12} and folic acid. Associated deficiencies of protein, pyridoxine, iron, and other substances involved in hematopoiesis undoubtedly play a role in this slow response.

Use of either vitamin B_{12} or folic acid alone therapeutically, without determination of the etiology of the megaloblastic anemia, cannot be condemned too strongly. Folic acid administration will often produce temporary hematologic remission, with eventual relapse, in the patient who is vitamin B_{12}-deficient, presumably through mobilization of the dwindling body stores of vitamin B_{12}.[71, 525-529] However, it has been repeatedly demonstrated that this procedure allows the development and progression of neurologic damage.[71, 525-527, 530-532]

Indeed, it has been suggested that folic acid administration may accelerate the speed of development of neurologic damage in the vitamin B_{12}-deficient patient. Both vitamin B_{12} and folic acid are involved in the synthesis of nucleic acids for blood formation [533] (see CHAPTER 3), but only vitamin B_{12} is required to maintain the integrity of the nervous system [423] (see CHAPTER 6). Administration of folic acid to the vitamin B_{12}-deficient patient produces a drop in the already low serum vitamin B_{12} level, which is proportional to the degree of the hematologic response,[534] and thereby presumably deprives the nervous system still further by drawing the body's small remaining vitamin B_{12} reserves into blood formation at the expense of the nervous system.[71]

In view of these facts, "shotgun" administration of multivitamin preparations and hematinics has rightly received strong condemnation.[13] Such preparations usually contain sufficient folic acid to support hematopoiesis and thereby mask the diagnosis of pernicious anemia, while allowing neurologic damage due to vitamin B_{12} deficiency to progress. Even as little as 0.3 mg. of folic acid, an amount which "will seldom support hematologic function in pernicious anemia," [535] may support such function when supplemented by the amount of folic acid in the patient's diet.

Particularly pernicious is the uncontrolled widespread public promotion and sale of "geriatric" vitamin preparations containing folic acid.[536] The sales campaigns for these preparations are aimed directly at the elderly part of the population, in which nearly all cases of pernicious anemia occur. The hapless victims of these campaigns are those individuals with vitamin B_{12} deficiency due to lack of intrinsic factor, who purchase with their geriatric vitamins an excellent chance for irreversible neurologic damage. Such sales are not controlled by law, and the promoters will not remove folic acid from their preparations for fear of not being able to compete with other "*complete* vitamin supplements."

Because of the seriousness of the neurologic damage which results from prolonged vitamin B_{12} deprivation, when the condition of the patient makes therapy necessary prior to establishment of the etiology of the megaloblastic anemia, vitamin B_{12} should be the initial therapeutic agent,[531] and should be given by injection.

In the folic acid-deficient patient, treatment with small doses of vitamin B_{12} may aggravate the clinical manifestations of the folic acid lack.[537] Severe, painful glossitis, atrophy of the lingual papillae, and cheilosis may develop or grow worse. It is not known whether the same phenomena may occur when large doses of vitamin B_{12} are used, but presumably they would.

In general terms, temporary hematologic remission in the vitamin B_{12}-deficient patient is more frequently accomplished with folic acid than is such remission in the folic acid-deprived patient when vitamin B_{12} is administered. Most B_{12}-deficient patients will sustain a temporary hematologic remission the first time they are given folic acid. The period of remission becomes shorter with each subsequent course of folic acid, until eventually the patient becomes totally refractory to this agent, with development of a hypocellular, nonmegaloblastic bone marrow and subsequently only a slow response to vitamin B_{12}, unassociated with a reticulocyte response.[71, 418]

Folic acid is unnecessary and unwarranted in the treatment of pure vitamin B_{12} deficiency states, such as that associated with pernicious anemia. It is true, however, that folic acid metabolism is interfered with in vitamin B_{12} deficiency. For example, folinic acid, rather than folic acid, is normally stored in the liver.[34, 39, 529] In vitamin B_{12} deficiency, however, a sizable portion of the liver store consists of folic acid.[34] This suggests that the ability to convert folic acid to folinic acid, and possibly to convert folic acid into any metabolically useful form, may depend in large part on the availability of vitamin B_{12}.

Subnormal "folic acid" levels have been found in the *whole blood* of some patients with pernicious anemia in relapse,[423] but *serum* "folic acid" levels have been normal in all such cases.[489] Other findings suggestive of possible folic acid deficiency in patients with pernicious anemia have included reduction in urinary excretion of folic acid before and shortly after vitamin B_{12} therapy, lowering of the blood folic acid levels following vitamin B_{12} injections, and rapid clearance of intravenously injected folic acid in some patients with untreated pernicious anemia.[304, 538]

In their review of folic acid and vitamin B_{12} interrelationships in pernicious anemia, supplemented by 12 years of their own studies, Will and his associates [71] point out that the various findings suggestive of associated folic acid deficiency in pernicious anemia are susceptible of other interpretations, primarily in terms of interference in folic acid metabolism due to lack of vitamin B_{12}. They observe that folic and folinic acid in serum may be used more rapidly in hematopoiesis, with tissue stores being used later, and that tissue depots may more avidly take up and retain folic and folinic acid when the vitamin B_{12} supply is inadequate.

Thus, while there is at present no direct evidence of inadequate stores of folic acid (although folinic acid stores may be depleted) in vitamin B_{12} deficiency states,[34] normal folic acid metabolism does appear to be dependent on an adequate supply of vitamin B_{12}, which may be involved in release of folinic acid from its tissue conjugates, facilitation of the reduction of folic acid to folinic acid, and in other biochemical mechanisms promoting the formation of N^{10}-formyl tetrahydrofolic acid,[71] currently believed to be the major active folic acid metabolite.[66]

In summary, there is probably no folic acid deficiency generally in patients with pernicious anemia in terms of *supply* of folic acid, but there is probably a folic acid deficiency in terms of *impaired utilization* of folic acid due to lack of vitamin B_{12}. Similar impaired utilization of folic acid probably occurs in all of the vitamin B_{12} deficiency states. The degree of impaired folic acid utilization is probably proportional to the degree of vitamin B_{12} deficiency.

Hematologic response of the folic acid-deficient patient to vitamin B_{12} administration is frequently incomplete, and may not occur at all. Almost every hematologist has had the experience of giving as much as 0.1 to 1 mg. of vitamin B_{12} to a patient with megaloblastic anemia and observing that the marrow remained megaloblastic. Such cases almost invariably turn out to be caused by folic acid deficiency, and respond dramatically to administration of this agent.

I. VITAMIN B_{12}

A. Parenteral

The only uniformly reliable way to administer vitamin B_{12} is by intramuscular or deep subcutaneous injection. The vitamin B_{12}-deficient patient requires sufficient vitamin B_{12} by this route of administration both to produce remission and to build up the depleted body stores of this vitamin.[34-36, 539] In this connection, it is an interesting fact that not all of the liver stores of vitamin B_{12} are available for blood formation. Patients with pernicious anemia may sometimes be noted to have a "spontaneous" remission if they develop hepatitis,[463, 464] which releases the liver vitamin B_{12} stores into the blood stream.[465, 540] It must be remembered that vitamin B_{12} is required wherever nucleo-protein synthesis is taking place, and this involves almost every tissue in the body, not only the hematopoietic and nervous systems.

A great deal of research has been devoted to an attempt to establish an ideal treatment schedule for the vitamin B_{12} defi-ciency states caused by inability to absorb the vitamin.[541–546] This work has shown that 90 to 95 per cent of an initial injected dose up to 50 μg. is retained, but the percentage retained of doses over this amount falls rapidly at a rate that is different for each patient.

Thus, within 48 hours after injections of 100 to 1000 μg. of vitamin B_{12}, from 50 to 98 per cent of the injected dose may appear in the urine,[543] although many patients may retain as much as 40 per cent of an initial 1000 μg. dose.[545.]

A single injection of 20 μg. of vitamin B_{12} will raise the serum level of a pernicious anemia patient to normal for about one to three weeks. The period for which serum B_{12} levels remain normal increases by smaller and smaller increments as the quan-tity of vitamin injected is increased, so that an injection of 160 μg. may keep the serum B_{12} normal for about two to seven weeks, and an injection of as much as 1000 μg. for only about five to eight weeks.[546]

These studies all indicated that the capacity of the serum and tissues to absorb vitamin B_{12} is limited to a certain maximum per unit time, and excess amounts of vitamin over this capacity are rapidly excreted. In addition, patients who lack intrinsic factor may have a reduced serum vitamin B_{12} binding capa-city,[547] although this has not yet been firmly established. This may be related to a possibly inadequate mechanism for storage of vitamin B_{12} which has not yet been demonstrated.[109, 206]

However, there are good arguments nonetheless in favor of initial therapy with large doses of vitamin B_{12}, and of mainte-nance with similar doses. (Vitamin B_{12} is nontoxic even when given in single doses as high as 3000 μg.[548, 549]) The vitamin B_{12}-

deficient patient achieves a normal serum B_{12} level with a single injection of less than 300 μg., but this level is in the low part of the normal range. Genuinely normal levels, in the range of the normal mean, are only achieved (after a single injection) when the amount injected is in excess of 300 μg.[546]

Resaturation of the body stores of vitamin B_{12} takes place more rapidly when large doses are given.[546] Recent studies suggest that even with such doses, resaturation is difficult to achieve within a three week period.[547]

Should future studies demonstrate that vitamin B_{12} is stored in the human liver as a B_{12} co-enzyme, as it may be in rabbit liver,[419a] such a B_{12} co-enzyme may prove to saturate the body stores more readily.

It has also been noted that a significant build-up in the vitamin B_{12} content of the spinal fluid can be obtained rapidly with daily injections of 1000 μg. of vitamin B_{12}.[543] This may be of significance in recovery from neurologic damage and in aborting further such damage, especially if "in contrast to other tissues, the brain takes up B_{12} more slowly, but shows a steady increment in the amount stored with continued injections."[550] In cases with neurologic involvement, it is not yet clear whether continuous administration of daily large doses of vitamin B_{12} is really more valuable than administration of moderate doses. Evaluation is complicated by difficulty in determining how much improvement is owing to the treatment itself and how much is owing to the frequent visits to the patient and testing of his dexterity and concern as to his mood.[551]

While 1 μg./day has been generally accepted as the "minimal maintenance requirement" for vitamin B_{12}, approximately 6 μg./day may prove a better estimate for optimal well-being of the patient.[552]

Keeping all of the above in mind, the most rational approach to therapy with vitamin B_{12} at the present time, in the private practice of medicine, is the administration of 1000 μg. of vitamin B_{12} (in 1 ml. of solution) every other day for a total of 5 doses as initial treatment to replenish substantially the body stores, followed by injection of 500 to 1000 μg./month as a maintenance dosage. The initial injections should be given every other day rather than every day because the percentage retention of each dose is substantially reduced if it is given only 24 hours after a prior dose.[541-546]

When there is neurologic damage, initial treatment should probably include 10 to 15 doses of 1000 μg. at daily intervals, followed by 1000 μg. once or twice weekly for several months, then gradual spacing of the interval between doses ending with 1000 μg. at monthly intervals after a period in excess of a year, when it appears no more neurologic recovery is likely to occur.[552a, 552b]

At some future date a reliable depot vitamin B_{12} preparation may be developed which will allow a longer interval between maintenance doses. An insoluble complex of vitamin B_{12}, zinc, and tannic acid is now being studied as such a repository preparation. Early reports mention no undesirable local or systemic effects due to the zinc or tannate.[553, 553a] Further evaluation is required to be certain such effects do not occur, and that the slowly released material is in fact vitamin B_{12} in a form available for human metabolism.

It is true that most patients can be maintained on monthly injections of vitamin B_{12} as low as 50 μg.[86] or 100 μg.,[554] but this may not always be adequate to maintain the body stores, and to maintain the patient in hematologic and neurologic remission in the face of any increased metabolic requirement or decreased capacity to respond to vitamin B_{12} such as accompanies illness. (A possible case in point[261] has been alluded to in the section, "Inability to Utilize Vitamin B_{12}.")

Maintenance therapy must continue for the lifetime of the patient who lacks intrinsic factor. This must be forcefully explained to the patient to prevent his "forgetting all about it" after the first injections of vitamin B_{12} produce a typical dramatic subjective and objective improvement. The patient who assumes after the first injections that he is cured often winds up in relapse with irreversible neurologic damage.

Because of the increased incidence of gastric cancer in patients with pernicious anemia, it may be wise to evaluate the patient at yearly intervals for a possible early gastric malignancy. Such evaluation may include roentgen studies as well as gastroscopy and microscopic study of gastric cells obtained by aspiration or by abrasive techniques.[555] It should certainly include thorough questioning of the patient for any symptoms of possible gastric origin. Such questioning is best done informally and without undue emphasis, to avoid cancerophobia.

Those few cases in which absorptive defect for vitamin B_{12} is correctible by surgery (structural abnormalities of the small intestine) may cease receiving maintenance therapy after such surgical correction and after demonstration that the ability to absorb vitamin B_{12} has been made normal is confirmed by a Schilling test, or another test of B_{12} absorption.

Patients whose vitamin B_{12} deficiency was due to dietary inadequacy or fish tapeworm may have their maintenance therapy terminated when their ingestion of vitamin B_{12} is adequate and anthelminthic therapy has expelled the worms. Before such termination, it should be determined by a Schilling test or other study that during the period of vitamin B_{12} deprivation the patient did not lose the ability to produce intrinsic factor because of gastric atrophy resulting from the vitamin deficiency.

B. Oral

Initiation of treatment for vitamin B_{12} deficiency should always be with parenteral administration of the vitamin. In the best circumstances, even in a normal gastrointestinal tract, absorption of vitamin B_{12} is extremely limited. It has not yet been demonstrated that it is possible to fill the depleted body stores of the B_{12}-deficient patient using any oral preparation.

Once repletion of the body stores has been accomplished by parenteral administration of vitamin B_{12}, one of the various oral preparations may be used for maintenance in certain selected patients, *provided the patients are carefully checked at regular intervals for any evidence of recurrent vitamin B_{12} defi-*

ciency. This should include thorough monthly examination of a peripheral blood smear for macroovalocytosis and an increase in the number of hypersegmented polymorphonuclear leukocytes, and complete neurologic examination. Where facilities for serum vitamin B_{12} determination are available, this should also be obtained at bimonthly intervals.

1. Vitamin B_{12} Alone

The absorption of physiologic (0.5 to 2 μg.) amounts of vitamin B_{12} is primarily dependent on the presence of intrinsic factor and a functionally normal small intestine. In a patient who lacks intrinsic factor and has megaloblastic anemia, any remission occurring while ingesting such doses (obtainable in a good diet) falls in the category of a "spontaneous" remission,[76, 260, 556] perhaps related in part to folic acid in the diet.

Oral maintenance therapy with physiologic doses of vitamin B_{12} is reserved exclusively for patients whose vitamin B_{12} deficiency was the result solely of inadequate ingestion of the vitamin, or a corrected inadequate absorption, uncomplicated by defective gastric secretion of intrinsic factor or malabsorption of vitamin B_{12}.

The absorption of supraphysiologic amounts of vitamin B_{12} is not intrinsic factor-dependent, and appears to take place by a mass action effect, possibly diffusion.[93-95, 112, 559, 560] About 1.5 μg. of a 50 μg. dose is absorbed mainly through this mechanism, and about 15 μg. of a 1000 μg. dose.[557]

Thus, some patients whose vitamin B_{12} deficiency was caused by inadequate or absent secretion of intrinsic factor and who have no small intestinal disorder may be maintained on small oral doses of as little as 15 to 50 μg. daily,[558] though relapse is frequent.[558a] Probably most patients may be marginally maintained by daily doses in excess of 100 μg.[96, 559, 560] Weekly single oral doses of 1000 μg. have been successful in maintaining a large group of such patients, but their serum vitamin B_{12} levels tend to be suboptimal, as do the serum levels of patients taking 50 μg. three times daily.[560] Therefore, oral maintenance with vitamin B_{12} at weekly intervals requires administration of more than 1000 μg. each week.[561, 562]

In general, oral treatment should not be employed if small intestinal dysfunction exists.

Oral treatment with vitamin B_{12} alone may be effective when the patient is very diligent in taking every dose of medication and returns at regular intervals no more than a month apart for thorough evaluation of his hematologic, neurologic, and general clinical status, preferably with determination of his serum vitamin B_{12} level as well. However, oral therapy with vitamin B_{12}, even in the best of circumstances, is not as reliable as parenteral therapy, and cannot be recommended.

2. Vitamin B_{12} Plus Hog Intrinsic Factor Concentrate

A priori, it would appear that ideal therapy for the patient who lacks intrinsic factor would be oral administration of the substance specifically lacking. This is especially true if intrinsic factor proves to be involved in vitamin B_{12} transport and storage, as may possibly be the case.[102–105, 108, 109, 206, 242, 563, 564] It is of great interest in this connection that the most active vitamin B_{12}-containing enzyme fraction of rat liver precipitates in 40 to 60 per cent ammonium sulfate,[432] which is almost identical to the 35 to 55 per cent ammonium sulfate concentration in which intrinsic factor precipitates.[119]

Concentrates of intrinsic factor derived from hog gastric, pyloric, and duodenal mucosa have been used successfully to maintain patients who lack intrinsic factor.[515, 565] However, an increasing number of cases have been reported in which maintenance therapy with some oral vitamin B_{12}-partially purified hog intrinsic factor combinations has been associated with development of inability of the patient to absorb the combined product, and eventual failure of such treatment.[260, 566–571] This phenomenon has not occurred to a great extent in two series of patients, however.[572, 573]

The evidence so far suggests that long term failure of oral therapy with heterologous preparations of partially purified hog intrinsic factor concentrate is due to development of resistance to some component of the concentrate. The "absorption block" may be partially or completely overcome by very large doses of concentrate.[570, 571, 574] Normal human gastric juice will still enhance vitamin B_{12} absorption after partially purified hog intrinsic factor concentrates fail.[566, 570] For some reason, relatively unpurified preparations of hog stomach and pyloric mucosa have not been associated with the development of resistance.[570]

Antibody to some component of hog intrinsic factor concentrates may develop in the blood of patients on prolonged oral vitamin B_{12}-intrinsic factor concentrate therapy,[575, 576] but no relation has been demonstrated between the presence of such antibody and refractoriness to such oral treatment.[575] It has not yet been determined whether this antibody is to intrinsic factor itself or to a contaminant in the concentrates. The antibody appears in vitro to precipitate human intrinsic factor concentrate as well as that from hogs,[575, 576] but whether the specific precipitate is intrinsic factor or another substance to which intrinsic factor loosely attaches has not been determined. A possible culprit may be blood group A substance, which is present in the most highly purified hog intrinsic factor concentrate currently available,[577] just as it is found in less purified concentrates.[578–581] Rabbits immunized to hog intrinsic factor concentrate [581a] (or to A substance?) do not produce anti-A agglutinins.

As has been suggested,[566] it is possible that a local antibody reaction to some component of heterologous intrinsic factor concentrate may develop at the hypothetical intestinal receptor site for intrinsic factor,[111, 112] resulting in rejection of such intrinsic factor.

At the present time, maintenance therapy with oral vitamin B_{12}-hog intrinsic factor concentrates (or concentrates from other animal species than man) should be used only with constant extreme vigilance against the development of refractoriness, including serial estimation of the vitamin B_{12} levels of serum.[260, 567] It is possible that pure intrinsic factor, when isolated, will be an oral therapeutic agent of choice. At present such treatment can not be recommended. The most recent work available [115a, 581b] suggests species specificity may be a problem with pure intrinsic factor.

3. Other Oral Therapies with Vitamin B_{12} and Added Agents

From time to time, a claim appears in the literature that vitamin B_{12} combined with one agent or another is or may be effective oral therapy for pernicious anemia.[582, 583] Such "improved oral therapies" usually turn out to depend for their effect primarily on their content of vitamin B_{12}, and offer no significant advantage over oral treatment with vitamin B_{12} alone.[559, 584-586]

A serious problem for the practicing physician as well as the public at large is the tremendous promotional campaign given almost every few months by many pharmaceutical firms to various combinations of vitamin B_{12} and any one of a number of agents which are said to enhance markedly vitamin B_{12} absorption. Any one of literally hundreds of agents taken orally may enhance absorption of vitamin B_{12} *by normal individuals,* but only intrinsic factor will generally enhance the absorption of vitamin B_{12} in the patient who lacks this agent. ACTH, steroids, or calcium in some cases, may improve intestinal absorption of vitamin B_{12} in patients with the malabsorption syndrome. The advertisements in medical journals of oral vitamin B_{12} combinations with this or that "miraculous absorption enhancement factor" adroitly omit any mention of the basic fact that the "miraculous absorption enhancement factor" may only work when the patient does not need treatment with vitamin B_{12} in the first place.

One such agent, d-sorbitol, is a hexahydric alcohol which may enhance the absorption of vitamin B_{12} in normal individuals [587] and in persons with normal baseline ability to absorb vitamin B_{12},[588] but not in patients unable to secrete intrinsic factor.[589] If it has any effect at all, which has been questioned,[590] it may act by stimulating gastric secretion of intrinsic factor,[591] and may be of use in a single very limited situation: that of the patient whose baseline secretion of intrinsic factor is low, but in whom administration of a secretagogue stimulates normal intrinsic factor output.[141, 588]

There are two immediately obvious mechanisms whereby an added agent may enhance vitamin B_{12} absorption in a normal subject: (1) by stimulating gastric secretion of intrinsic factor, and (2) by combining with vitamin B_{12} in a bond which is only broken in the alkaline medium of the small intestine. The latter mechanism is effective because, for unknown reasons, vitamin B_{12} which bypasses the stomach is better absorbed than vitamin B_{12} which passes through the stomach in uncombined form.[174-176] Other mechanisms may exist, but they are as yet undefined.

The only way the practicing physician can protect his patients from useless oral "therapies" is to ignore the pharmaceutical firm advertisements that flood his mail and his medical journals and rely on treatment that he knows has stood the test of time. The physician should realize that just because many of these oral "therapies" are promoted only on an "ethical" basis, i.e., only to physicians, such promotion is no guarantee of efficacy.

Other than for their content of vitamin B_{12} alone, oral therapy with vitamin B_{12} and the various "absorption-enhancing agents" has no place in the treatment of megaloblastic anemias, at the present time.

II. FOLIC ACID

Folic acid, in oral doses of 5 to 10 mg. daily, is effective in the treatment of most cases of folic acid deficiency.[592, 593] An occasional refractory patient may require a larger dose,[286] but such patients may suffer from multiple deficiencies and require correction of such deficiencies rather than larger doses of folic acid. Cases in point are those with ascorbic acid deficiency.

It is noteworthy that even in those patients whose folic acid deficiency is due to impaired absorption of the vitamin, oral therapy with 5 to 10 mg. daily doses is effective. Such doses are probably considerably in excess of the minimal daily requirement for this vitamin, and may pass whatever intestinal barrier may exist to folic acid absorption by a mass action effect. It is also possible that unconjugated folic acid is absorbed with relative ease, whereas the folic acid conjugates present in food may be absorbed with greater difficulty, or may have to be deconjugated prior to absorption.

It is of interest that patients with idiopathic steatorrhea who have been on adrenal steroid therapy for many years may have persistently low serum "folic acid" levels with macrocytosis and an Arneth count "shift to the right" despite ingestion of 0.25 mg. of folic acid three times daily. This suggests that the persistence of jejunal mucosal damage is accompanied by persistence of inability to absorb physiologic doses of folic acid (i.e., doses in the range of 0.5 mg. or less).

Parenteral administration of folic acid may be required in the presence of severe diarrhea, and in megaloblastic anemia in infancy, if there is difficulty in giving the vitamin perorally. Generally, the dose given parenterally is as large as that given by mouth, but doses of 1 mg. of folic acid are adequate when injected to produce remission. Repletion of body stores of folic acid may require larger doses, but these may usually be given subsequently by mouth.

Maintenance therapy, after repletion of the body stores, may be carried out with as little as 0.25 to 0.5 mg. of folic acid daily, and a good diet. The latter alone is generally effective in supplying an adequate amount of folic acid. In severe malabsorption syndromes, however, 5 to 10 mg. daily by mouth may be required because of persistent inability to absorb physiologic doses.

III. CITROVORUM FACTOR (FOLINIC ACID)

The one specific indication for citrovorum factor therapy, in doses of 3 to 6 mg., is to overcome the effects of the folic acid antagonists employed in cancer chemotherapy.[594] These agents, such as Aminopterin, both compete with and irreversibly block the conversion of folic acid to its metabolically useful form, for periods of two to three weeks after administration.[350, 595]

While they also compete with citrovorum factor, which is formed in the body from folic acid and convertible to the same active form as is folic acid,[596] they do not block its utilization.[350, 351, 593]

IV. LIVER EXTRACT

It is unlikely that liver extract has any therapeutic usefulness not due to its content of vitamin B_{12} and folic acid. Liver extract has many disadvantages as a therapeutic agent when compared to the pure vitamins: it is more costly, less concentrated, more likely to produce pain at injection sites, and may produce allergic reactions.[86, 597]

While it is possible that another as yet not isolated factor may be present in liver extract that may be effective in a rare case of megaloblastic anemia unresponsive to vitamin B_{12} or folic acid,[598] no such factor has yet been defined.

It has been claimed[599, 600] that there is a "protein synthesis" factor present in liver extracts which is neither vitamin B_{12} nor folic acid. The claim was based on two observations, neither of which has been confirmed by most other observers. First, it was stated that reduced prothrombin times generally occur in patients with pernicious anemia and related macrocytic anemias, and that liver extracts more rapidly restore such reduced prothrombin times to normal than either vitamin B_{12} or folic acid. Second, it was stated that liver extract restored macrocytosis to normocytosis more efficiently than vitamin B_{12} or folic acid.

It is possible that in pernicious anemia liver stores of agents other than vitamin B_{12} and folic acid are disturbed. There is usually an irregular pattern of liver dysfunction in pernicious anemia.[462] As to the possible need for liver extract to restore prothrombin time to normal, reduction in prothrombin time sometimes occurs in association with pernicious anemia,[601] but this phenomenon may well be the exception rather than the rule.[384] It may be related to the anorexia, nausea, and vomiting of untreated patients.[602] When it occurs, it is restored to normal after adequate specific therapy with vitamin B_{12} alone. The hemorrhagic manifestations sometimes seen in untreated pernicious anemia are, in the author's experience, uniformly associated with thrombocytopenia which clears on specific therapy, and only irregularly associated with reduced prothrombin time.

Perhaps the claim of a "protein synthesis" factor arose in part from inclusion of patients with the malabsorption syndrome. Such patients frequently not only absorb vitamin B_{12} and folic acid poorly, thereby developing a megaloblastic anemia, but also have grossly impaired absorption of vitamin K for synthesis of prothrombin and other "serum factors" involved in blood clotting.[603, 604] In these patients, injection of vitamin K_1 rapidly restores prothrombin, Factor VII, and Stuart factor to normal.[603] Here, too, no specific value of liver extract over adequate vitamin B_{12}, folic acid, and vitamin K administration has been documented.

There is no objective evidence for the claim that liver extracts restore macrocytosis to normocytosis more rapidly than equivalent amounts of vitamin B_{12} and folic acid. Treatment of the megaloblastic anemias with adequate specific therapy is generally efficient in eliminating all vestiges of the anemia, including the macrocytosis. Two to four months of therapy are usually required.

V. ASCORBIC ACID (Vitamin C)

The patient with megaloblastic anemia due at least in part to ascorbic acid deficiency should receive about 2 Gm. of vitamin C by mouth to resaturate his tissues, administered in divided doses of 100 mg. five times a day.[605-607] An equal amount may be given parenterally if the patient can not take oral medication. Within 24 hours on this regimen any active bleeding ceases. After this, maintenance therapy consists of 200 mg. per day until recovery is assured, and 100 mg. daily thereafter. The above doses may be halved for infants.[607] The maintenance requirement for ascorbic acid in infants is met by ingesting orange juice regularly, and in children and adults, by ingesting a well balanced diet including citrus fruits, tomatoes, and vegetables.

Various workers have suggested an interrelationship between ascorbic acid and cyanocobalamin because untreated patients with megaloblastic anemia often have low serum ascorbic acid levels, and intravenously administered ascorbic acid disappears more rapidly in the vitamin B_{12}-deficient patient than it does in the normal subject.[608, 609] However, "the nature of the association of B_{12} deficiency and the abnormality of ascorbic acid metabolism is by no means clear though it is evident that the latter plays no fundamental part in the production of a megaloblastic anemia in B_{12} deficiency." [608] Treatment of nearly all megaloblastic anemias, except perhaps some of the megaloblastic anemias of infancy and the rare cases that may occur with scurvy, does not require the use of ascorbic acid, nor does such use have any known value.

In this conection, it should be noted that the finding of *any ascorbic acid at all* in plasma or whole blood is incompatible with a diagnosis of scurvy unless the vitamin has recently been administered.[381] A level up to 4 mg. per cent in the buffy coat of the blood is compatible with scurvy, however.[605]

VI. BLOOD TRANSFUSION

"When the initial hematocrit is below 15 per cent, particularly in elderly persons, a single transfusion, preferably of packed red cells, is advisable to sustain the patient until response to vitamin B_{12} (or folic acid) can occur." [86] In the patient with dehydration associated with the malabsorption syndrome, whole blood transfusion is preferable unless congestive heart failure is present. In the absence of a very low hematocrit, or serious complicating factors such as infections or cardiac disorders, it is rarely necessary to transfuse patients with megaloblastic anemia, since the response to specific therapy is rapid enough to restore the hematologic status to normal in a short time.

It must be emphasized that, even with a hematocrit below 15 per cent or a hemoglobin below 5 Gm./100 ml. of blood, more than one transfusion is rarely either needed or desirable. It is deplorable that so many unnecessarily panic-stricken physicians give not one transfusion but so many that circulatory overload may result,[536] the patient is unnecessarily endangered,[610] and the hematologic response to therapy is masked. For these physicians, a few quotes from Crosby's editorial, in the journal "Blood," on the misuse of blood transfusion,[610] may be in order: "Anemia alone is not a sufficient justification" for transfusion. "Most bedfast patients are comfortable with as little as 5 or 6 grams" of hemoglobin. "The dangers of blood transfusion, infection, hemosiderosis, and transfusion reaction are well known. . . . Thoughtless prescription of blood transfusion is playing Russian roulette with bottles of blood instead of a revolver."

VII. ADRENOCORTICOTROPHIC HORMONE (ACTH) AND ADRENOCORTICAL STEROIDS

ACTH or the adrenocortical steroids will often correct the absorptive defect for vitamin B_{12} associated with tropical sprue,[207, 213, 214] and are useful in the management of that disease and often of other disorders presenting with the clinical picture of the malabsorption syndrome,[611, 612] including regional ileitis.[229] They did not correct the absorptive defect for vitamin B_{12} in nontropical sprue, in most of the cases seen by the author.

Hematologic response to adrenocortical steroid therapy has been observed in some cases of addisonian pernicious anemia and of adult coeliac disease, in 2 cases of rheumatoid arthritis associated with megaloblastic anemia and a low serum vitamin B_{12} level despite normal vitamin B_{12} absorption, and 1 case of megaloblastic anemia after partial gastrectomy.[214, 215] In only 1 case, a patient with addisonian pernicious anemia,[215] was the absorption of vitamin B_{12} enhanced during the steroid therapy; in that case intrinsic factor secretion did not appear to have been enhanced despite the hematologic response. The mechanism of action of the steroid therapy in these few cases is unknown, and the hematologic response is generally slow when it occurs at all. For these reasons, steroids are not considered to have a place in the treatment of megaloblastic anemias other than those associated with generalized severe malabsorption.

VIII. OTHER THERAPY

Treatment other than as outlined above would depend on the condition causing the megaloblastic anemia. Such treatment would include insuring an adequate diet in all cases and a gluten-free diet in childhood and adult coeliac disease [219, 224]; prescribing anthelminthics in cases of fish tapeworm infestation; appropriate antibiotics in the blind loop syndrome; surgery where feasible to correct structural abnormalities of the small intestine; and correction of endocrine disorders. In addition, appropriate supportive measures are self evident, as is prompt and vigorous antibiotic therapy in old patients with pernicious anemia in relapse who develop pneumonia or urinary tract infections.[536] The key to such treatment is accurate differential diagnosis of the cause of the megaloblastic anemia, supplemented by thorough evaluation of the patient for any related or unrelated disorders.

Summary

THE LITERATURE on the megaloblastic anemias has been reviewed, with special emphasis on recent advances in knowledge, and supplemented by the author's experiences and research with patients and in the laboratory. The megaloblastic anemias have been discussed in terms of their incidence, hematologic morphology, biochemical basis, etiologic classification, clinical picture, differential diagnosis, and therapy.

The heart of this monograph has been the presentation of the etiologic classification of the megaloblastic anemias. They are seen to be primarily due to inadequate ingestion, absorption, or utilization of vitamin B_{12} or folic acid. The possible causes in each case are presented.

Clear understanding of the possible causes of each of these inadequacies forms the basis for accurate differential diagnosis, and, in turn, of proper and specific treatment of each case.

Rapid and accurate recognition, differential diagnosis, and treatment of a patient with a megaloblastic anemia frequently provide the richest reward in the practice of medicine: achievement of an almost overnight transformation from a moribund, seemingly hopeless state to one of vigor, health, and vitality.

References

1. EHRLICH, P.: De- und Regeneration roter Blutscheiben. Verhandl. deutsch Gesellsch. d. Char., (June 10 and Dec. 9) 1880.
2. REISNER, E. H., JR.: The nature and significance of megaloblastic blood formation. Blood 13:313, 1958.
3. MOLLIN, D. L.: Radioactive vitamin B_{12} in the study of blood diseases. Brit. M. Bull. 15:8, 1959.
4. GIRDWOOD, R. H.: The role of folic acid in the blood disorders. Brit. M. Bull. 15:14, 1959.
5. WILLS, L.: Pernicious anemia, nutritional macrocytic anemia, and tropical sprue: a discussion. Blood 3:36, 1948.
6. ——: Studies in pernicious anemia of pregnancy. VI. Tropical macrocytic anemia as a deficiency disease, with special reference to the vitamin B complex. Indian J. M. Res. 21:699, 1934.
7. FOY, H., KONDI, A., AND SAEMA, B.: The anemias of the tropics, India, and Ceylon. J. Trop. Med. 61:27, 1958; Tr. Roy. Soc. Trop. Med. & Hyg. 52:46, 1958.
8. DAS GUPTA, C. R., AND CHATTERJEA, J. B.: The role of synthetic folic acid (L. casei factor) in the treatment of nutritional macrocytic anemia. Ind. M. Gaz. 81:402, 1946.
9. FAIRLEY, N. H., BROMFIELD, R. J., FOY, H., AND KONDI, A.: Nutritional macrocytic anemia in Macedonia. A preliminary report. Tr. Roy. Trop. Med. & Hyg. 32:132, 1938.
10. TASKER, P. W. G., MOLLIN, D. L., AND BERRIMAN, H.: Vitamin B_{12} deficiency in the megaloblastic anemias of Malaya. Brit. J. Haemat. 4:167, 1958.
11. TOTTERMAN, G.: On the occurrence of pernicious tapeworm anemia in Diphyllobothrium carriers. Acta med. scandinav. 118:410, 1944.
12. FRIEDLANDER, R. D.: Racial factor in pernicious anemia. Am. J. M. Sc. 187:634, 1934.
13. WINTROBE, M. M.: Clinical Hematology. Philadelphia, Lea & Febiger, 1956.
13a. BINGHAM, J. The macrocytosis of hepatic disease. I. Thin macrocytosis. Blood 14:694, 1959.
14. NORDENSON, N. G., SEGERDAHL, E. STRANDELL, B., AND WALLMAN-CARLSSON, C.: Die Frequenz und geographische Verbreitung der pernizösen Anämie in Schweden. Acta med. scandinav. 97:222, 1938.
15. REISNER, E. H., JR., WOLFF, J. A., McKAY, R. J., JR., AND DOYLE, E. F.: Juvenile pernicious anemia. Pediatrics. 8:88, 1951.
16. EDITORIAL: Age and vitamin B_{12} metabolism. Nutrit. Rev. 17:40, 1959.
17. KRISTENSEN, H. P. O., AND GORMSEN, H.: Vitamin B_{12} deficiency in uncharacteristic macrocytic anemia. Comparison of bone marrow findings and vitamin B_{12} levels in plasma. Acta med. scandinav. 162:415, 1958.
18. TAUBER, S. A., GOODHART, R. S., HSU, J. M., BLUMBERG, N., KASSAB, J., AND CHOW, B. F.: Vitamin B_{12} deficiency in the aged. Geriatrics 12:368, 1957.

19. JONES, O. P.: Origin of neutrophils in pernicious anemia (Cooke's macro-polycytes). Arch. Int. Med. *60*:1002, 1937.

20. ARNETH, J.: Qualitativ Blutlehre und Blutkrankheiten. Leipzig, J. A. Barth, 1945.

21. WINTROBE, M. M.: Diagnostic significance of changes in leucocytes. Bull. New York Acad. Med. *15*:223, 1939.

22. STORTI, E.: Diagnostic des Maladies du Sang, translated into French by J. Targhetta, and A Daumas. Paris, G. Doin, 1959.

23. ARNETH, J.: Über das qualitativ Verhalten der Blutplättchen bei der Perniciösa. Folia haemat. *57*:1, 1937.

24. FINCH, C. A., COLEMAN, D. H., MOTULSKY, A. G., DONOHUE, D. M., AND REIFF, R. H.: Erythrokinetics in pernicious anemia. Blood *11*:807, 1956.

25. CAZAL, P.: Erythrocytes et Erythropathies. Paris, Masson, 1957.

26. MALLARMÉ, J.: The study of the myelogram in pernicious anemia and the problem of the megaloblast. Blood *3*:103, 1948.

27. ——, AND DEBRAY, J.: Les Anémies Mégaloblastiques. Paris, S.E.P.E.S., 1949.

28. BESSIS, M.: Cytology of the Blood and Blood-Forming Organs, translated into English by E. Ponder. New York, Grune & Stratton, 1956.

29. REISNER, E. H., JR., AND KORSON, R.: Microspectrophotometric determination of desoxyribosenucleic acid in megaloblasts of pernicious anemia. Blood *6*:344, 1951.

30. PAULSON, M., AND HARVEY, J. C.: Hematologic alterations after total gas-trectomy: evolutionary sequence over a decade. J.A.M.A. *156*:1556, 1954.

31. DARBY, W. J., BRIDGFORTH, E. B., LE BROCQUEY, J., CLARK, S. L., JR., DE OLIVEIRA, J. D., KEVANY, J., McGANITY, W. J., AND PEREZ, C.: Vitamin B_{12} requirement of adult man. Am. J. Med. *25*:726, 1958.

32. BOEN, S. T., MOLHUYSEN, J. A., AND STEENBERGEN, J.: Nuclear changes in oral epithelial cells in subacute combined degeneration of the spinal cord due to vitamin-B_{12} deficiency. Lancet *2*:294, 1958.

33. HOLMES, J. M.: Cerebral manifestation of vitamin B_{12} deficiency. Brit. M. J. *2*:1394, 1956.

34. GIRDWOOD, R. H.: The occurrence of growth factors for lactobacillus leish-manii, streptococcus faecalis, and leuconostoc citrovorum in the tissues of pernicious anemia patients and controls. Biochem. J. *52*:58, 1952.

35. SWENDSEID, M. E., HVOLLBOLL, E., SCHICK, G., AND HALSTED, J. A.: The vitamin B_{12} content of human liver tisssue and its nutritional significance; a com-parison study of various age groups. Blood *12*:24, 1957.

36. GLASS, G. B. J.: Radioactive vitamin B_{12} in the liver. III. Hepatic storage and discharge of $CO^{60}B_{12}$ in pernicious anemia. J. Lab. & Clin. Med. *52*:875, 1958.

37. SCHLOESSER, L. L., DESHPANDE, P., AND SCHILLING, R. F.: Biological turnover rate of cyanocobalamin (vitamin B_{12}) in human liver. Arch. Int. Med. *101*:306, 1958.

38. GLASS, G. B. J.: Deposition and storage of vitamin B_{12} in the normal and diseased liver. Gastroenterology *36*:180, 1959. Paper discussed by: Halsted, J. A., Popper, H., and Heinrich, H. C.

39. SWENDSEID, M. E., BETHELL, F. H., AND ACKERMANN, W. W.: The intracellular distribution of vitamin B₁₂ and folinic acid in mouse liver. J. Biol. Chem. *190*:791, 1951.

40. HERBERT, V., STORER, J., AND SPAET, T. H.: Unpublished data.

41. UNDRITZ, E.: Sandoz Atlas of Haematology. Basle, Frobenius, 1952.

42. WEICKER, H.: Hämo-Zytomorphologie des B₁₂-Mangels in vivo. *In* Heinrich, H. C.: Vitamin B₁₂ und Intrinsic Factor. Stuttgart, Ferdinand Enke, 1957.

43. FUDENBERG, H., AND ESTREN, S.: Non-addisonian megaloblastic anemia. The intermediate megaloblast in the differential diagnosis of pernicious and related anemias. Am. J. Med. *25*:198, 1958.

44. DACIE, J. V.: Discussion. Brit. M. J. *1*:702, 1948.

45. EDITORIAL: The intermediate megaloblast. Lancet *1*:105, 1959.

46. MOLLIN, D. L.: The intermediate megaloblast. Brit. M. J. *1*:302, 1959.

47. DACIE, J. V., AND WHITE, J. C.: Erythropoiesis with particular reference to its study by biopsy of human bone marrow. A review. J. Clin. Path. *2*:1, 1949.

48. BARBIER, F.: Un cas particulier d'hypersegmentation constitutionelle des noyaux des neutrophiles chez l'homme. Acta haemat. *19*:121, 1958.

48a. PEDERSON, J., LUND, J., OHLSEN, A. S., AND KRISTENSEN, H. P. O.: Simultaneous deficiency of iron and vitamin B₁₂. Dimorphic anemia. Acta med. scandinav. *163*:235, 1959.

49. TROWELL. H. C.: Dimorphic anaemia: deficiency of iron associated with nutritional macrocytic anaemia. Tr. Roy. Soc. Trop. Med. & Hyg. *37*:18, 1943.

50. THEORELL, B.: Studies on the formation of cellular substances during blood production. Acta med. scandinav. (suppl. 200) *129*, 1947.

51. ——: The relation of nucleic acid to the formation and differentiation of cellular proteins. Cold Spring Harbor Symposia on Quant. Biol. *12*:247, 1948.

52. WHITE, J. C., LESLIE, I., AND DAVIDSON, J. N.: Nucleic acids of bone marrow cells, with special reference to pernicious anemia. J. Path. & Bact. *66*:291, 1953.

53. MUELLER, J. F., GLAZER, H. S., AND VILTER, R. W.: Preliminary studies on the purine and pyrimidine bases of human bone marrow as determined by paper chromatography. I. Variations in pernicious anemia in response to therapy. J. Clin. Invest. *31*:651, 1952.

54. FRIEDKIN, M., AND WOOD, H.: Conversion of uracil deoxyriboside to thymidine of deoxyribosenucleic acid. J. Biol. Chem. *220*:645, 1956.

54a. SMITH, L. H., JR., AND BAKER, F.: Pyrimidine studies in pernicious anemia. J. Clin. Invest. *38*:1044, 1959.

55. CASTLE, W. B.: Development of knowledge concerning the gastric intrinsic factor and its relation to pernicious anemia. New England J. Med. *249*:603, 1953.

56. GRAHAM, R. M., AND RHEAULT, M. H.: Characteristic cellular changes in cells of nonhemopoietic origin in pernicious anemia. J. Lab. & Clin. Med. *43*:235, 1954.

57. MASSEY, B. W., AND RUBIN, C. E.: The stomach in pernicious anemia. Am. J. M. Sci. 227:481, 1954.

58. BOEN, S. T.: Changes in epithelial cells in vitamin B_{12} deficiency. In Heinrich, H. C.: Vitamin B_{12} und Intrinsic Factor. Stuttgart, Ferdinand Enke, 1957.

59. GARDNER, F. H.: Observations on the cytology of gastric epithelium in tropical sprue. J. Lab. & Clin. Med. 47:529, 1956.

60. JACOBSON, W.: The mode of action of folic acid antagonists and the function of the Leuconostoc Citrovorum factor. In Wolstenholme, G. E. W., and Cameron, M. P.: Ciba Foundation Symposium on Chemistry and Biology of Pteridines. Boston, Little, Brown & Co., 1954.

61. STOKSTAD, E. L. R.: Some properties of a growth factor for lactobacillus casei. J. Biol. Chem. 149:573, 1943.

62. PFIFFNER, P. J., BINKLEY, S. B., BLOOM, E. S., BROWN, R. A. BIRD, O. D., AND EMMETT, A. D.: Isolation of the anti-anemia factor (vitamin B_c) in crystalline form from liver. Science 97:404, 1943.

63. RICKES, E. L., BRINK, N. G., KONIUSZY, F. R., WOOD, T. R., AND FOLKERS, K.: Crystalline vitamin B_{12}. Science 107:396, 1948.

64. SMITH, E. L.: Purification of anti-pernicious anemia factors from liver. Nature 161:638, 1948.

65. ARNSTEIN, H. R. V.: The function of vitamin B_{12} and folic acid in the metabolism of one-carbon units. In Heinrich, H. C.: Vitamin B_{12} und Intrinsic Factor. Stuttgart, Ferdinand Enke, 1957.

66. BROQUIST, H. P.: Water-soluble vitamins, part I (folic acid, B_{12} group, choline). Ann. Rev. Biochem. 27:285, 1958.

67. ARNSTEIN, H. R. V.: The function of vitamin B_{12} in animal metabolism. Biochem. Soc. Symposia 13:92, 1955.

68. SHIVE, W.: The functions of B-vitamins in the biosynthesis of purines and pyrimidines. Vitamins & Hormones 9:75, 1951.

69. JUKES, T. H., AND STOKSTAD, E. L. R.: The role of vitamin B_{12} in metabolic processes. Vitamins & Hormones 9:1, 1951.

70. FORD, J. E., AND HUTNER, S. H.: Role of vitamin B_{12} in the metabolism of microorganisms. Vitamins & Hormones 13:101, 1955.

70a. RUNDLES, R. W.: Hematopoietic effects of folic acid metabolites in the megaloblastic anemias. Am. J. Clin. Nutrition. 7:385, 1959.

71. WILL, J. J., MUELLER, J. F., BRODINE, C., KIELY, C. E., FRIEDMAN, B., HAWKINS, R. N., DUTRA, J., AND VILTER, R. W.: Folic acid and vitamin B_{12} in pernicious anemia. J. Lab. & Clin. Med. 53:22, 1959.

72. SMITH, E. L.: Vitamin B_{12}. Brit. M. Bull. 12:52, 1956.

73. THOMAS, E. D., AND LOCHTE, H. L., JR.: Studies on the biochemical defect of pernicious anemia. I. In vitro observations on oxygen consumption, heme synthesis and deoxyribonucleic acid synthesis by pernicious anemia bone marrow. J. Clin. Invest. 37:166, 1958.

74. HALL, B. E., AND CAMPBELL, D. C.: Vitamin B_{12} therapy in pernicious anemia. I. Effect on hematopoietic system: preliminary report. II. Effect on the general clinical and neurologic manifestations: preliminary report. Proc. Staff Meet. Mayo Clin. 23:584, 1948; 23:591, 1948.

75. BETHELL, F. H., MEYERS, M. C., AND NELIGH, R. B.: Vitamin B_{12} in pernicious anemia and puerperal macrocytic anemia. J. Lab. & Clin. Med. *33*:477, 1948.

76. DARBY, W. J., JONES, E., CLARK, S. L., McGANITY, W. J., DE OLIVEIRA, J. D., PEREZ, C., KEVANY, J., AND LE BROCQUY, J.: The development of vitamin B_{12} deficiency by untreated patients with pernicious anemia. Am. J. Clin. Nutrition. *6*:513, 1958.

77. JUKES, T. H., AND WILLIAMS, W. L.: Occurrence of vitamin B_{12} in food. *In* Sebrell, W. H., and Harris, R. S.: The Vitamins, New York, Academic Press, 1954, vol. 1.

78. LEWIS, U. J., REGISTER, U. D., THOMPSON, H. T., AND ELVEHJEM, C. A.: Distribution of vitamin B_{12} in natural materials. Proc. Soc. Exper. Biol. & Med. *72*:479, 1949.

79. KARLIN, R.: La vitamine B_{12} dans le lait humain et bovin. Compt. rend. Soc. de biol. *148*:371, 1954.

80. WOKES, F., BADENOCH, J., AND SINCLAIR, H. M.: Human dietary deficiency of vitamin B_{12}. Am. J. Clin. Nutrition. *3*:375, 1955.

81. GOUNELLE, H., AND RICHARD, J.: Low serum vitamin B_{12} concentrations in alcoholics; improvement with liver therapy. Am. J. Clin. Nutrition. *6*:422 1958.

82. MOVITT, E. R.: Megaloblastic erythropoiesis in patients with cirrhosis of the liver. Blood *5*:468, 1950.

83. WATSON, J., LICHTMAN, H. C., MESSITE, J., ELLISON, R. R., CONRAD, H., AND GINSBERG, V.: Clinical studies with the citrovorum factor in megaloblastic anemia. Am. J. Med. *17*:17, 1954.

84. JANDL, J. H., AND LEAR, A. A.: The metabolism of folic acid in cirrhosis. Ann. Int. Med. *45*:1027, 1956.

85. WELLS, R.: Nutritional vitamin B_{12} deficiency. J. Trop. Med. *61*:81, 1958.

86. McINTYRE, P., KREVANS, J. R., AND CONLEY, C. L.: Treatment of megaloblastic anemias. J. Chron. Dis. *6*:287, 1957.

87. POLLYCOVE, M., APT, L., AND COLBERT, M. J.: Pernicious anemia due to dietary deficiency of vitamin B_{12}. New England J. Med. *255*:164, 1956.

88. ANDRUS, E. C., AND WINTROBE, M. M.: Hyperthyroidism and pernicious anemia. Bull. Johns Hopkins Hosp. *59*:291, 1936.

89. BOENHEIM, F., SCHWIMER, D., AND McGAVACK, T. H.: The combination of hyperthyroidism and pernicious anemia. Ann. Int. Med. *27*:869, 1945.

90. ZIFFER, H., GUTMAN, A., PASHER, I., SOBOTKA, H., AND BAKER, H.: Vit. B_{12} in thyrotoxicosis and myxedema. Proc. Soc. Exper. Biol. & Med. *96*:229, 1957.

91. GERSHOFF, S. N., VITALE, J. J., ANTONOWICZ, I., NAKAMURA, M., AND HELLERSTEIN, E. E.: Studies of interrelationships of thyroxine, magnesium, and vitamin B_{12}. J. Biol. Chem. *231*:849, 1958.

92. FORSSELL, J., AND HALONEN, P. I.: Thyroid function and pernicious anemia. Acta med. scandinav. *162*:61, 1958.

93. ROSS, G. I. M., MOLLIN, D. L., COX, E. V., AND UNGLEY, C. C.: Hematologic

responses and concentration of vitamin B₁₂ in the serum and urine following oral administration of vitamin B₁₂ without intrinsic factor. Blood *9:*473, 1954.

94. UNGLAUB, W. G., ROSENTHAL, H. L., AND GOLDSMITH, G. A.: Studies of vitamin B₁₂ in serum and urine following oral and parenteral administration. J. Lab. & Clin. Med. *43:*143, 1954.

95. DOSCHERHOLMEN, A., AND HAGEN, P. S.: A dual mechanism of vitamin B₁₂ plasma absorption. J. Clin. Invest. *36:*1551, 1957.

96. ESTREN, S., BRODY, E. A., AND WASSERMAN, L. R.: The metabolism of vitamin B₁₂ in pernicious and other megaloblastic anemias. Advances Int. Med. *9:*11, 1958.

97. BAKER, S. J., AND MOLLIN, D. L.: The relationship between intrinsic factor and the intestinal absorption of vitamin B₁₂. Brit. J. Haemat. *1:*46, 1955.

98. ADDISON, T.: On the constitutional and local effects of disease of the suprarenal capsules. London, S. Highley, 1855. See also ADDISON, T.: Anemia—disease of the suprarenal capsules. Lond. Med. Gaz. *43:*517, 1849.

99. BIERMER, A.: Über progressiv perniciöse Anämie. Korresp. schweiz. Ärzte *2:*15, 1872.

100. VON BONSDORFF, B.: Pathogenesis of vitamin B₁₂ deficiency, with special reference to tapeworm pernicious anemia. *In* Heinrich, H. C.: Vitamin B₁₂ und Intrinsic Factor. Stuttgart, Ferdinand Enke, 1957.

101. MINOT, G. R., AND MURPHY, W. P.: Treatment of pernicious anemia by a special diet. J.A.M.A. *87:*470, 1926.

102. CASTLE, W. B.: Observations on the etiologic relationship of achylia gastrica to pernicious anemia. I. The effect of the administration to patients with pernicious anemia of the contents of the normal human stomach recovered after the ingestion of beef muscle. Am. J. M. Sci. *178:*748, 1929.

103. ——, AND TOWNSEND, W. C.: *Ibid.* II. The effect of the administration to patients with pernicious anemia of beef muscle after incubation with normal human gastric juice. Am. J. M. Sci. *178:*764, 1929.

104. ——, ——, AND HEATH, C. W.: *Ibid.* III. The nature of the reaction between normal human gastric juice and beef muscle leading to clinical improvement and increased blood formation similar to the effect of liver feeding. Am. J. M. Sci. *180:*305, 1930.

105. ——, HEATH, C. W., AND STRAUSS, M. B.: *Ibid.* IV. A biologic assay of the gastric secretion of patients with pernicious anemia having free hydrochloric acid and that of patients without anemia or with hypochromic anemia having no free hydrochloric acid, and of the role of intestinal impermeability to hematopoietic substances in pernicious anemia. Am. J. M. Sci. *182:*741, 1931.

106. BERK, L., CASTLE, W. B., WELCH, A. D., HEINLE, R. W., ANKER, R., AND EPSTEIN, M.: *Ibid.* X. Activity of vitamin B₁₂ as food (extrinsic) factor. New England J. Med. *239:*911, 1948.

107. GARDNER, F. H., HARRIS, J. W., SCHILLING, R. F., AND CASTLE, W. B.: *Ibid.* XI. Hematopoietic activity in pernicious anemia of a beef muscle extraction

containing food (extrinsic) factor upon intravenous injection without contact with gastric (intrinsic) factor. J. Lab. & Clin. Med. *34:*1502, 1949.

108. HERBERT, V.: In vitro organ specificity of intrinsic factor action. Fed. Proc. *17:*440, 1958.

109. ——, AND SPAET, T. H.: Distribution of "intrinsic factor" action. Am. J. Physiol. *195:*194, 1958.

110. ——: On the mechanism of action of intrinsic factor. Presented to Montefiore Hosp. Research Soc., December 20, 1957.

111. ——: Mechanism of intrinsic factor action in the isolated rat small intestine. J. Clin. Invest. *37:*901, 1958.

112. ——: Mechanism of intrinsic factor action in everted sacs of rat small intestine. J. Clin. Invest. *38:*102, 1959.

113. TAYLOR, K. B., MALLETT, B. J., AND SPRAY, G. H.: Observations on the inhibitory effects of intrinsic factor preparations on vitamin B_{12} absorption. Clin. Sc. *17:*647, 1958.

114. ——: Personal communication.

115. ABELS, J.: Intrinsic Factor van Castle en Resorptie van Vitamine B_{12}. Doctoral Thesis, University of Groningen. Groningen, V. R. B., March 11, 1959.

115a. COOPER, B. A., AND CASTLE, W. B.: Factors influencing the action of intrinsic factor in vivo. Clinical Research *7:*206, 1959.

116. LATNER, A. L. AND MERRILLS, R. J.: Further observations related to the isolation of intrinsic factor mucoprotein. *In* Heinrich, H. C.: Vitamin B_{12} und Intrinsic Factor. Stuttgart, Ferdinand Enke, 1957.

117. WILLIAMS, W. L., AND ELLENBOGEN, L.: Purification and assay of intrinsic factor. *In* Heinrich, H. C.: Vitamin B_{12} und Intrinsic Factor. Stuttgart, Ferdinand Enke, 1957.

118. GLASS, G. B. J., BOYD, L. J., RUBINSTEIN, M. A., AND SVIGALS, C. S.: Relationship of glandular mucoprotein from human gastric juice to Castle's intrinsic anti-anemia factor. Science *115:*101, 1952.

119. WIJMENGA, H. G.: Intrinsic factor and vitamin B_{12}-binding substances. Purification, properties, and possible relationship. *In* Heinrich, H. C.: Vitamin B_{12} und Intrinsic Factor. Stuttgart, Ferdinand Enke, 1957.

120. FOX, H. J., AND CASTLE, W. B.: Observations on the etiologic relationship of achylia gastrica to pernicious anemia. IX. Difference in site of secretion of intrinsic factor in the hog and in the human stomach. Am. J. M. Sc. *203:*18, 1942.

121. LANDBOE-CHRISTENSEN, E., AND PLUM, C. M.: Experimental study on the localization of Castle's intrinsic factor in the human stomach. Anti-anemic effect of powdered human fundus and pylorus. Am. J. M. Sc. *215:*17, 1948; *ibid. 224:*1, 1952; Acta med. scandinav. *144:*467, 1953; *ibid. 150:*369, 1954.

122. KEUNING, F. J., ARENDS, A., MANDEMA, E., AND NIEWIG, H. O.: Observations on the site of production of Castle's intrinsic factor in the rat. J. Lab. & Clin. Med. *53:*127, 1959.

123. MOLLIN, D. L., BAKER, S. J., AND DONIACH, I.: Addisonian pernicious anemia without gastric atrophy in a young man. Brit. J. Haemat. *1:*278, 1955.

124. FENWICK, S.: On atrophy of the stomach. Lancet *2:*78, 1870.

125. MAGNUS, H. A.: A re-assessment of the gastric lesion in pernicious anemia. J. Clin. Path. *11:*289, 1958.

126. GLASS, G. B. J.: Gastric atrophy. Its clinical significance and methods of detection. Am. J. Digest. Dis. *2:*709, 1957.

127. SIURALA, M.: Gastric lesion in some megaloblastic anemias. Acta med. scandinav. *154:*337, 1956.

128. DAVIDSON, W. M. B., AND MARKSON, J. L.: The gastric mucosa in iron deficiency anemia. Lancet *2:*639, 1955.

129. WITTS, L. J.: Simple achlorhydric anemia. Guy's Hosp. Rep. *80:*253, 1930.

130. STEVENSON, T. D., LITTLE, J. A., AND LANGELY, L.: Pernicious anemia in childhood. New England J. Med. *255:*1219, 1956.

131. FINNEY, J. O.: Pernicious anemia unassociated with achlorhydria. Ann. Int. Med. *12:*1521, 1939.

132. ASKEY, J. M.: Addisonian pernicious anemia without achlorhydria: does it exist? Gastroenterology *2:*1, 1944.

133. JACOBS, A.: Acid secretion by the stomach in pernicious anemia. Brit. J. Haemat. *4:*465, 1958.

134. MACLACHLAN, W. W. G., AND KLINE, F. M.: Occurrence of anemia in 4 generations. Am. J. M. Sci. *172:*533, 1926.

135. CALLENDER, S. T., AND DENBOROUGH, M. A.: A family study of pernicious anemia. Brit. J. Haemat. *3:*88, 1957.

136. McINTYRE, P. A., HAHN, R., CONLEY, C. L., AND GLASS, B.: Genetic factors in predisposition to pernicious anemia. Bull. Johns Hopkins Hosp. *104:*309, 1959.

137. ARBO, J., AND MOHR, J.: Pernicious anemia in monovular twins. Acta genet. et stat. med. *8:*105, 1958.

138. HARRIS-JONES, J. N., SWAN, H. T., AND TUDHOPE, G. R.: Pernicious anemia without gastric atrophy and in the presence of free hydrochloric acid: report of a case. Blood *12:*461, 1957.

139. BAKER, S. J., AND MOLLIN, D. L.: The relationship between intrinsic factor and vitamin B_{12} absorption. Rev. hémat. *10:*180, 1955.

140. MOLLIN, D. L., BOOTH, C. C., AND BAKER, S. J.: The absorption of vitamin B_{12} in control subjects, in addisonian pernicious anemia and in the malabsorption syndrome. Brit. J. Haemat. *3:*412, 1957.

141. LEE, S., HERBERT, V., AND WASSERMAN, L. R.: Unpublished case report.

142. GOLDHAMER, S. M.: The presence of the intrinsic factor of Castle in the gastric juice of patients with pernicious anemia. Am. J. M. Sc. *191:*405, 1936.

143. EDITORIAL: Heredity in gastric cancer and pernicious anemia. Lancet *2:*1215, 1954.

144. MOSBECH, J.: Heredity in Pernicious Anemia. Copenhagen, Ejnar Munksgaard, 1953.

145. UNGLEY, C. C.: Some current views on the origin of pernicious anemia and the absorption of vitamin B_{12}. Tr. New York Acad. Sc. *14:*25, 1951.

146. CONNOR, H. M.: Hereditary aspect of achlorhydria in pernicious anemia. J.A.M.A. *94:*606, 1930.

147. WILLIAMS, A. W., COGHILL, N. F., AND EDWARDS, F.: The gastric mucosa in pernicious anemia: biopsy studies. Brit. J. Haemat. *4*:457, 1958.

148. FABER, K.: The etiology and pathogenesis of achylia gastrica. *In* Lectures in Internal Medicine. New York, Paul B. Hoeber, 1927.

149. JOSKE, R. A., FINCKH, E. S., AND WOOD, I. J.: Gastric biopsy: a study of 1,000 consecutive successful gastric biopsies. Quart. J. Med. *24*:269, 1955.

150. ALSTED, G.: Pernicious anemia after nitric acid corrosion of the stomach. Lancet *1*:76, 1937.

151. BEYERS, M. R., DIEFENBACH, W. C. L., MARK, H., AND MEYER, L. M.: Interrelationship of folic acid and vitamin B_{12} in macrocytic anemia associated with linitis plastica. Acta med. scandinav. *142*:351, 1952.

152. GOLDHAMER, S. M.: Macrocytic anemia in carcinoma of the stomach apparently due to lack of intrinsic factor. Am. J. M. Sc. *195*:17, 1938.

153. KAPLAN, H. S., AND RIGLER, L. G.: Pernicious anemia and carcinoma of the stomach: autopsy studies concerning their relationship. Am. J. M. Sc. *209*:339, 1945.

154. MOSBECH, J., AND VIDEBAEK, A.: Mortality from and risk of gastric carcinoma among patients with pernicious anemia. Brit. M. J. *2*:390, 1950.

155. ZAMCHEK, N., GRABLE, E., LEY, A., AND NORMAN, L.: Occurrence of gastric cancer among patients with pernicious anemia at the Boston City Hospital. New England J. Med. *252*:1103, 1955.

156. SNAPPER, I., GROEN, J., HUNTER, D., AND WITTS, L. J.: Achlorhydria, anemia, and subacute combined degeneration in pituitary and gonadal insufficiency. Quart. J. Med. *6*:195, 1937; Lancet *2*:307, 1942.

157. LEITHOLD, S. L., DAVID, D., AND BEST, W. R.: Hypothyroidism with anemia demonstrating abnormal vitamin B_{12} absorption. Am. J. Med. *24*:535, 1958.

158. HERBERT, V.: Unpublished data.

159. BOENHEIM, F.: Addison's disease and pernicious anemia. Endokrinologie *28*:140, 1951.

160. BERLIN, R.: Addison's disease: familial incidence and occurrence in association with pernicious anemia. Acta med. scandinav. *144*:1, 1952.

161. PAULSEN, M., CONLEY, C. L., AND GLADSDEN, E. S.: Absence of intrinsic factor from intestinal juice of patients following total gastrectomy. Am. J. M. Sc. *220*:310, 1950.

162. McLEAN, L. D.: Incidence of megaloblastic anemia after subtotal gastrectomy. New England J. Med. *257*:262, 1957.

163. LOEWENSTEIN, F.: Absorption of cobalt[60]-labeled vitamin B_{12} after subtotal gastrectomy. Blood *13*:339, 1958.

164. BADENOCH, J., EVANS, J. R., RICHARDS, W. C. D., AND WITTS, L. J.: Megaloblastic anemia following partial gastrectomy and gastroenterostomy. Brit. J. Haemat. *1*:339, 1955.

165. BRODINE, C., FRIEDMAN, B. I. SAENGER, E. L., AND WILL, J. J.: The absorption of vitamin B_{12} labeled with radioactive cobalt[60] following subtotal gastrectomy. J. Lab. & Clin. Med. 53:220, 1959.

165a. FORSHAW, J. W. B.: Hyperproteinaemia after partial gastrectomy corrected by gluten-free diet. Brit. Med. J. *2*:1020, 1958.

165b. LUNDH, G.: Intestinal digestion and absorption after gastrectomy. Acta chirurg. scandinav. (Suppl. 231) 1958.

166. BROWN, E. B., Jr., AND JUSTUS, B. W.: In vitro absorption of radioiron by everted pouches of rat intestine. Am. J. Physiol. 194:319, 1958.

166a. MOORE, C. V., AND DUBACH, R.: Resorption, conservation, elimination, and physiological iron losses. In Keiderling, W., Ed.: Eisenstoffwechsel. Stuttgart, G. Thieme, 1959.

167. BADENOCH, J., EVANS, J. R., AND RICHARDS, W. C. D.: The stomach in hypochromic anaemia. Brit. J. Haemat. 3:175, 1957.

168. LI, J. G., METTIER, S. R., HARPER, H. A., AND McBRIDE, A.: Pernicious anemia due to the presence of intrinsic factor inhibitor diagnosed in childhood, with a 25-year follow-up. Clinical Research 7:90, 1959.

169. GLASS, G. B. J., BOYD, L. J., STEPHANSON, L., AND JONES, E. L.: Metabolic interrelations between intrinsic factor and vit. B_{12}. III. B_{12} absorption at varied intrinsic factor doses. Proc. Soc. Exper. Biol. & Med. 88:1, 1955.

170. CALLENDER, S. T., AND EVANS, J. R.: Observations on the relationship of intrinsic factor to the absorption of labelled vitamin B_{12} from the intestine. Clin. Sc. 14:387, 1955.

171. TAYLOR, K. B., MALLETT, B. J., WITTS, L. J., AND TAYLOR, W. H.: Observations on vitamin B_{12} absorption in the rat. Brit. J. Haemat. 4:63, 1958.

172. WILLIAMS, W. L., CHOW, B. F., ELLENBOGEN, L., AND OKUDA, K.: Intrinsic factor preparations which augment and inhibit absorption of vitamin B_{12} in healthy individuals. In Heinrich, H. C.: Vitamin B_{12} und Intrinsic Ftcor. Stuttgart, Ferdinand Enke, 1957.

173. GOLDSMITH, G. A.: Nutritional anemias with especial reference to vitamin B_{12}. Am. J. Med. 25:680, 1958.

173a. HERBERT, V., CASTRO, Z., AND WASSERMAN, L. R.: Unpublished data.

174. CITRIN, Y., DeROSA, C., AND HALSTED, J. A.: Sites of absorption of vitamin B_{12}. J. Lab. & Clin. Med. 50:667, 1957.

175. HALSTED, J. A., GASSTER, M., AND DRENICK, E. J.: Absorption of radioactive vitamin B_{12} after total gastrectomy. New England J. Med. 251:161, 1954.

176. JOHNSON, P. C., AND BERGER, E. S.: Enhanced urinary excretion of Co^{60} vitamin B_{12} produced by delayed release capsules. Blood 13:457, 1958.

177. BIRD, O. D., AND HOEVET, B.: The vitamin B_{12}-binding power of proteins. J. Biol. Chem. 190:181, 1951.

178. BAURIEDEL, W. R., PICKEN, J. C., Jr., AND UNDERKOFLER, L. A.: Reactions of cyanocobalamin and aquocobalamin with proteins. Proc. Soc. Exper. Biol. & Med. 91:377, 1956.

179. GRÄSBECK, R.: Studies on the vitamin B_{12}-binding principle and other biocolloids of human gastric juice. Acta med. scandinav., Suppl. 314, 1956.

180. CASTLE, W. B., HEATH, C. W., STRAUSS, M. B., AND HEINLE, R. W.: Observations on the etiologic relationship of achylia gastrica to pernicious anemia. VI. Site of interaction of food and gastric factors: failure of in vivo incubation to produce thermostable hematopoietic principle. Am. J. M. Sc. 194:618, 1937.

181. McIntyre, P. A., Sachs, M. V., Krevans, J. R., and Conley, C. L.: Pathogenesis and treatment of macrocytic anemia. Information obtained with radioactive vitamin B_{12}. Arch. Int. Med. 98:541, 1956.

182. Booth, C. C., and Mollin, D. L.: The site of absorption of vitamin B_{12} in man. Lancet 1:18, 1959.

183. Latner, A. L.: Intrinsic factor and vitamin B_{12} absorption. Brit. M. J. 2:278, 1958.

184. Reynell, P. C., Spray, G. H., and Taylor, K. B.: The site of absorption of vitamin B_{12} in the rat. Clin. Sc. 16:663, 1957.

185. Herbert, V., Castro, Z., and Wasserman, L. R.: Localization of the effect of intrinsic factor in the rat small intestine in vitro. Clinical Research 7:33, 1959.

186. Baker, S. J., Mackinnon, N. L., and Vasudevia, P.: Site of absorption of orally administered vitamin B_{12} in dogs. Indian J. M. Res. 46:812, 1958.

187. Callender, S. T., and Spray, G. H.: Preparation of haemopoietically active extracts from faeces. Lancet 1:1391, 1951.

188. Ross, G. I. M., and Mollin, D. L.: Vitamin B_{12} in tissues in pernicious anemia and other conditions. In Heinrich, H. C.: Vitamin B_{12} und Intrinsic Factor. Stuttgart, Ferdinand Enke, 1957.

189. Ellenbogen, L., and Williams, W. L.: Personal communication. See Tables 9 and 10.

190. Glass, G. B. J.: Differentiation of macrocytic anemias and detection of a pernicious anemia and sprue in remission by accelerated measurement of hepatic uptake of radioactive Co^{60}-B_{12}. In Proceedings of the Sixth International Congress of the International Society of Hematology. New York, Grune & Stratton, 1958.

191. Oxenhorn, S., Estren, S., Wasserman, L. R., and Adlersberg, D.: Malabsorption syndrome: intestinal absorption of vitamin B_{12}. Ann. Int. Med. 48:30, 1958.

192. Cooke, W. T.: The malabsorption syndrome in man: Pathogenesis—current concepts. National Vitamin Foundation Symposium, March 3, 1959. Am. J. Clin. Nutrition. (in press).

193. Adlersberg, D.: The malabsorption syndrome in man: Clinical and pathological aspects. National Vitamin Foundation Symposium, March 3, 1959. Am. J. Clin. Nutrition. (in press).

194. Gardner, F. H.: The malabsorption syndrome in man: Hematologic aspects. National Vitamin Foundation Symposium, March 3, 1959. Am. J. Clin. Nutrition. (in press).

195. French, A. B.: The malabsorption syndrome in man: Management. National Vitamin Foundation Symposium, March 3, 1959, Am. J. Clin. Nutrition. (in press).

196. Panel and Open Discussion: The malabsorption syndrome in man. National Vitamin Foundation Symposium, March 3, 1959. Am. J. Clin. Nutrition. (in press).

197. Adlersberg, D., Wang, C. I., and Bossak, E. T.: Disturbance in protein and lipid metabolism in malabsorption syndrome. J. Mount Sinai Hosp. (New

York) 24:206, 1957. Simultaneously published in Adlersberg, D.: The Malabsorption Syndrome. New York, Grune & Stratton, 1957.

198. PATERSON, J. C. S.: The sprue syndrome. Am. J. M. Sc. 231:92, 1956.

199. HUNTER, F. M., AND PREVATT, A. L.: Diagnostic methods in intestinal malabsorption. Am. J. M. Sc. 236:81, 1958.

199a. VOLWILER, W.: Gastrointestinal Malabsorptive Syndromes. Chicago, Year Book Publishers, 1959.

200. HIMES, H. W., AND ADLERSBERG, D.: Pathologic changes in the small bowel in idiopathic sprue; biopsy and autopsy findings. Gastroenterology 35:142, 1958.

201. SHINER, M.: Small intestinal biopsies by the oral route. Histopathologic changes in the malabsorption syndrome. J. Mount Sinai Hosp. (New York) 24:273, 1957. Simultaneously published in Adlersberg, D.: The Malabsorption Syndrome. New York, Grune & Stratton, 1957.

202. SMITH, R. B. W., SPRINZ, H., CROSBY, W. H., AND SULLIVAN, B. H.: Peroral small bowel mucosal biopsy. Am. J. Med. 25:391, 1958.

203. SHINER, M.: Conference: Anaemia and the alimentary tract. Lancet 2:255, 1958.

204. COOKE, W. T.: Adult coeliac disease and other disorders associated with steatorrhea. Brit. M. J. 2:261, 1958.

205. BUTTERWORTH, C. E., AND PEREZ-SANTIAGO, E.: Jejunal biopsies in sprue. Ann. Int. Med. 48:8, 1958.

206. HERBERT, V.: Studies on the role of intrinsic factor in vitamin B_{12} absorption, transport, and storage. Symposium on Vitamin Interrelationships, Medical College of Virginia, Richmond, October 24, 1958. Am. J. Clin. Nutrition. 7:433, 1959.

207. FROST, J. W., GOLDWEIN, M. I., AND KAUFMAN, B.: Studies of B_{12}-CO^{60} absorption in malabsorption syndrome: results before and during specific therapy. Ann. Int. Med. 47:293, 1957.

208. JOSKE, R. A., SHAMMA'A, M. H., AND DRUMMEY, G. D.: Intestinal malabsorption following temporary occlusion of the superior mesenteric artery. Am. J. Med. 25:449, 1958.

209. GRASBECK, R., KANTERO, I., AND SIURALA, M.: Influence of calcium ions on vitamin B_{12} absorption in steatorrhea and pernicious anemia. Lancet 1:234, 1959.

210. ASHFORD, B. K.: Sprue. In Tice's Practice of Medicine. Hagerstown, Md., W. F. Prior, vol. 4, p. 173.

211. SPIES, T. D., MILANES, F., MENENDEZ, A., KOCH, M. B., AND MINNICH, V.: Observations on the treatment of tropical sprue with folic acid. J. Lab. & Clin. Med. 31:227, 1946.

212. STEFANINI, M.: Clinical features and pathogenesis of tropical sprue. Medicine 27:379, 1948.

213. GLASS, G. B. J.: Intestinal absorption and hepatic uptake of vitamin B_{12} in diseases of the gastrointestinal tract. Gastroenterology 30:37, 1956.

214. DOIG, A., GIRDWOOD, R. H., DUTHIE, J. J. R., AND KNOX, J. D. E.: Response of megaloblastic anemia to prednisolone. Lancet 2:966, 1957.

215. FROST, J. W., AND GOLDWEIN, M. I.: Observations on vitamin B_{12} absorption in primary pernicious anemia during administration of adrenocortical steroids. New England J. Med. 258:1096, 1958.

216. KEELE, K. D.: The prognosis and treatment of sprue in India. Brit. M. J. 1:986, 1949.

217. HAZARI, O. K., AND WOODRUFF, A. W.: Prognosis of tropical sprue. Brit. M. J. 2:344, 1958.

218. COMBINED STAFF CLINIC: Malabsorption syndrome. Am. J. Med. 15:790, 1953.

219. FRENCH, J. M., AND HAWKINS, C. F.: The gluten-free diet in idiopathic steatorrhea. Med. Clin. North American 41:1585, 1957.

219a. SCHWARTZ, M. K., SLEISENGER, M. P., PERT, J. H., ROBERTS, K. E., RANDALL, H. T., AND ALMY, T. P.: The effect of a gluten-free diet on fat, nitrogen, and mineral metabolism in patients with sprue. Gastroenterology 32:232, 1957.

220. THAYSEN, T. E. H.: Non-Tropical Sprue. London, Oxford University Press, 1932.

221. ADLERSBERG, D.: Introduction to symposium on the malabsorption syndrome. J. Mount Sinai Hosp. (New York) 24:177, 1957. Simultaneously published in Adlersberg, D.: The Malabsorption Syndrome. New York, Grune & Stratton, 1957.

222. RUBIN, C. E., BRANDBORG, L. L., PHELPS, P. C., AND TAYLOR, H. C., JR.: Intestinal similarities between celiac disease and idiopathic sprue. J. Clin. Invest. 37:927, 1958.

223. ——, ——, AND ——: Is the intestinal pathology of celiac disease reversible? A preliminary report. Clinical Research 7:120, 1959.

224. FRENCH, J. M., HAWKINS, C. F., AND SMITH, N.: The effect of a wheat-gluten-free diet in adult idiopathic steatorrhoea. Quart. J. Med. 26:481, 1957.

225. KELLEY, M. L., AND TERRY, R.: Clinical and histological observations in fatal non-tropical sprue. Am. J. Med. 25:460, 1958.

226. THOMPSON, M. W.: Heredity, maternal age, birth order in etiology of celiac disease. Am. J. Human Genet. 3:159, 1951.

227. DAVIDSON, L. S. P., AND FOUNTAIN, J. R.: Incidence of sprue syndrome with some observations on natural history. Brit. M. J. 1:1157, 1950.

228. ANDERSON, D. H., AND DiSANT'AGNESE, P. A.: Idiopathic celiac disease. I. Mode of onset and diagnosis. Pediatrics 11:207, 1953.

229. COOKE, W. T.: Conference: Anaemia and the alimentary tract. Lancet 2:255, 1958.

230. PLUM, P., AND WARBURG, E.: Hematological changes, especially megalocytic anemia in regional ileitis. Acta med. scandinav. 102:449, 1939.

231. CAMERON, D. G., WATSON, G. M., AND WITTS, L. J.: Clinical association of macrocytic anemia with intestinal stricture and anastomoses. Blood 4:793, 1949.

232. THOMPSON, R. B., AND UNGLEY, C. C.: Megaloblastic anemia associated with anatomic lesions in the small intestine. Blood 10:771, 1955.

233. HALSTED, J. A., LEWIS, P. M., AND GASSTER, M.: Absorption of radioactive

vitamin B_{12} in the syndrome of megaloblastic anemia associated with intestinal stricture or anastomosis. Am. J. Med. 20:42, 1956.

234. KOGAN, E., SCHAPIRA, A., JANOWITZ, H. D., AND ADLERSBERG, D.: Malabsorption following extensive small intestinal resection including inadvertent gastro-ileostomy. J. Mount Sinai Hosp. (New York) 24:399, 1957. Simultaneously published in Adlersberg, D.: The Malabsorption Syndrome. New York, Grune & Stratton, 1957.

235. HARRISON, H. E., HARRISON, H. C., TOMPSETT, R. R., AND BARR, D. P.: Potassium deficiency in a case of lymphosarcoma with the sprue syndrome. Am. J. Med. 2:131, 1947.

236. BJERKELUND, C. J.: Symptomatic sprue. Acta med. scandinav. 137:130, 1950.

237. HENDRIX, J. P., BLACK-SCHAFFER, B., WITHERS, R. W., AND HANDLER, P.: Whipple's intestinal lipodystrophy. Arch. Int. Med. 85:91, 1950.

238. OXENHORN, S., ESTREN, S., AND ADLERSBERG, D.: Intestinal uptake of vitamin B_{12} in the malabsorption syndrome. J. Mount Sinai Hosp. (New York) 24:232, 1957. Simultaneously published in Adlersberg, D.: The Malabsorption Syndrome. New York, Grune & Stratton, 1957.

239. BRUGSCH, H.: Hyperchromic anemia in chronic disorders of pancreas. Arch. f. klin. Med. 173:199, 1932.

240. KEEFER, C. S., HUANG, K. K., AND YANG, C. S.: Anemia associated with chronic dysentery. Arch. Int. Med. 47:436, 1931.

241. OKUDA, K.: Vitamin B_{12} metabolism and thyroid hormones. Nisshim Igaku 45:331, 1958.

242. HERBERT, V.: Studies of intrinsic factor mechanism of action. Vitamin B_{12} Symposium, New York Medical College, April 11, 1958 (in press).

243. GRÄSBECK, R., AND NYBERG, W.: Inhibition of radiovitamin B_{12} absorption by ethylenediaminetetraacetate (EDTA) and its reversal by calcium ions. Scandinav. J. Clin. & Lab. Invest. 10:448, 1958.

244. HENNEMAN, P. H., BENEDICT, P. H., FORBES, A. P., AND DUDLEY, H. R.: Idiopathic hypercalcuria. New England J. Med. 259:802, 1958.

245. REISNER, E. H., JR., GILBERT, J. P., ROSENBLUM, C., AND MORGAN, M. C.: Applications of the urinary tracer test (of Schilling) as an index of vitamin B_{12} absorption. Am. J. Clin. Nutrition. 4:134, 1956.

245a. RUBIN, C. E.: Personal communication.

246. BRANTE, G., AND ERNBERG, T.: The in vitro uptake of vitamin B_{12} by Diphyllobothrium latum and its blockage by intrinsic factor. Scandinav. J. Clin. & Lab. Invest. 9:313, 1957.

247. NYBERG, W.: The absorption of radioactive vitamin B_{12} in persons infested with the fish tapeworm, Diphyllobothrium latum. In Heinrich, H. C.: Vitamin B_{12} und Intrinsic Factor. Stuttgart, Ferdinand Enke, 1957.

248. BRANTE, G., AND ERNBERG, T.: The mechanism of pernicious tapeworm anemia studied with Co60-labeled vitamin B_{12}. Acta med. scandinav. 160:91, 1958.

249. VON BONSDORFF, B.: Pernicious anemia caused by Diphyllobothrium latum, in the light of recent investigations. Blood 3:91, 1948; Acta med. scandinav. 144:263, 1953.

250. BADENOCH, J.: The blind loop syndrome. *In* Jones, F. A.: Modern Trends in Gastroenterology. New York, Paul Hoeber, 1958.

251. SIURALA, M., AND KAIPANEN, W. J.: Intestinal megaloblastic anemia, treated with aureomycin and terramycin. Acta med. scandinav. *147:*197, 1953.

252. BADENOCH, J., BEDFORD, P. D., AND EVANS, J. R.: Massive diverticulosis of the small intestine with steatorrhoea and megaloblastic anemia. Quart. J. Med. *24:*321, 1955.

253. BURKHOLDER, P. R.: Microbiological studies on materials which potentiate oral vitamin B$_{12}$ therapy in addisonian anemia. Arch. Biochem. *39:*322, 1952.

254. SYDERHELM, R., LEHMANN, W., AND WICHELS, P.: Experimentelle intestinale perniziose Anämie beim Hund. Klin. Wchnschr. *2:*1439, 1924.

255. CAMERON, D. G., WATSON, G. M., AND WITTS, L. J.: The experimental production of macrocytic anemia by operations on the intestinal tract. Blood *4:*803, 1949.

256. WATSON, G. M., AND WITTS, L. J.: Intestinal macrocytic anemia. Brit. M. J. *1:*13, 1952.

257. LICHTMAN, H., GINSBERG, V., AND WATSON, J.: Therapeutic effect of aureomycin in pernicious anemia. Proc. Soc. Exper. Biol. & Med. *74:*884, 1950.

258. FOY, H., AND KONDI, A.: The haematinic action of penicillin in megaloblastic anemia and its relationship to B$_{12}$ metabolism and the intestinal flora. Tr. Roy. Soc. Trop. Med. & Hyg. *48:*17, 1954.

259. GIRDWOOD, R. H.: The megaloblastic anemias. Quart. J. Med. *25:*87, 1956.

260. KILLANDER, A.: Oral treatment of pernicious anemia with vitamin B$_{12}$ and purified intrinsic factor. I. The value of serial estimation of the vitamin B$_{12}$ levels of serum. Acta med. scandinav. *160:*339, 1958.

261. HERBERT, V., WASSERMAN, M., AND SPAET, T. H.: Unpublished case report.

262. WAGLE, S. R., MEHTA, R., AND JOHNSON, B. C.: Vitamin B$_{12}$ and protein biosynthesis. V. The site of action of vitamin B$_{12}$ and its inhibition by a B$_{12}$ antagonist. Biochim. et biophys. acta *28:*215, 1958.

263. MULGAONKAR, A. G., AND SREENIVASAN, A.: Alterations in rat serum proteins in folic acid and vitamin B$_{12}$ deficiencies. Proc. Soc. Exper. Biol. & Med. *94:*44, 1957.

264. BAKER, H., FRANK, O., PASHER, I., HUTNER, S., HERBERT, V., AND SOBOTKA, H.: Substituted vitamin B$_{12}$ amides. I. A microbiologic study. Proc. Soc. Exper. Biol. & Med. *100:*825, 1959.

265. HERBERT, V., HOOGSTRATEN, B., BAKER, H., AND WASSERMAN, L. R.: Patients given prolonged treatment with substituted amides of vitamin B$_{12}$ in an attempt to control neoplastic growth. Unpublished cases.

266. OKUDA, K., HELLEGERS, A. E., AND CHOW, B. F.: Vitamin B$_{12}$ serum level and pregnancy. Am. J. Clin. Nutrition. *4:*440, 1956.

267. BAKER, H., ERDBERG, R., PASHER, I., AND SOBOTKA, H.: Study of folic acid and vit. B$_{12}$ in blood and urine during normal pregnancy. Proc. Soc. Exper. Biol. & Med. *94:*513, 1957.

268. BOGER, W. P., BAYNE, G. M., WRIGHT, L. D., AND BECK, G. D.: Differential

serum vitamin B_{12} concentrations in mothers and infants. New England J. Med. *256*:1085, 1957.

269. PRYSTOWSKY, H., HELLEGERS, A. E., RANKE, E., RANKE, B., AND CHOW, B. F.: Further observations on the metabolism of vitamin B_{12} in human pregnancy. Am. J. Obst. & Gynec. *77*:1, 1959.

269a. BAKER, H., ZIFFER, H., PASHER, I., AND SOBOTKA, H.: A comparison of maternal and foetal folic acid and vitamin B_{12} at parturition. Brit. M. J. *1*:978, 1958.

270. HELLEGERS, A., OKUDA, K., NESBITT, R. E. L., JR., SMITH, D. W., AND CHOW, B. F.: Vitamin B_{12} absorption in pregnancy and in the newborn. Am. J. Clin. Nutrition. *5*:327, 1957.

271. LUHBY, A. L., COOPERMAN, J. M., DONNENFELD, A. M., HERRERO, J. M., TELLER, D. N., AND WENIG, J. B.: Observations on transfer of vitamin B_{12} from mother to fetus and newborn. Proc. Soc. Pediatric Res., 28th Annual Meeting, p. 140, (May 6–7) 1958; A.M.A. J. Dis. Child. *96*:532, 1958.

272. HUNT, J. N., AND MURRAY, F. A.: Gastric function in pregnancy. J. Obst. & Gynaec. Brit. Emp. *65*:78, 1958.

273. GILES, C., AND SHUTTLEWORTH, E. M.: Megaloblastic anaemia of pregnancy and the puerperium. Lancet *2*:1341, 1958.

274. IZAK, G., RACHMILEWITZ, M., STEIN, Y., BERKOVICI, B., SADOVSKY, A., ARONOVITCH, Y., AND GROSSOWICZ, N.: Vitamin B_{12} and iron deficiencies in anemia of pregnancy and puerperium. Arch. Int. Med. *99*:346, 1957.

275. HEINRICH, H. C.: Die biochemischen Grundlagen der Diagnostik und Therapie der Vitamin B_{12}-Mangelzustände (B_{12}-Hypo- und Avitaminosen) des Menschen und der Haustiere: Untersuchungen zum Vitamin B_{12} Stoffwechsel des Menchen während der Gravidität und Lactation. Klin. Wchnschr. *32*:205, 1954.

276. CALLENDER, S. T. E.: A critical review of pernicious anemia of pregnancy. Quart. J. Med. *13*:75, 1944.

277. DAS GUPTA, C. R., CHATTERJEA, J. B., AND BASU, P.: Vitamin B_{12} in macrocytic anaemia in pregnancy. Indian M. Gaz. *88*:102, 1953; Indian J. M. Res. *42*:411, 1954.

278. ISRAELS, M. C. G., AND DA CUNHA, F. A. L.: Megaloblastic anaemia of pregnancy. Lancet *2*:214, 1952.

279. BADENOCH, J., CALLENDER, S. T., EVANS, J. R., TURNBULL, A. L., AND WITTS, L. J.: Megaloblastic anaemia of pregnancy and the puerperium. Brit. M. J. *1*:1245, 1955.

280. MOLLIN, D. L., AND ROSS, G. I. M.: Vitamin B_{12} deficiency in the megaloblastic anaemias. Proc. Roy. Soc. Med. *47*:428, 1954.

281. LOWENSTEIN, L., PICK, C., AND PHILPOTT, M.: Megaloblastic anemia of pregnancy and the puerperium. Am. J. Obst. & Gynec. *70*:1309, 1955.

282. PITNEY, W. R., BEARD, M. F., AND VAN LOON, E. J.: Observations on the bound form of vitamin B_{12} in human serum. J. Biol. Chem. *207*:143, 1954.

283. MENDELSOHN, R. S., WATKIN, D. M., HORBETT, A. P., AND FAHEY, J. L.: Identification of the vitamin B_{12}-binding protein in the serum of normals and of patients with chronic myelocytic leukemia. Blood *13*:740, 1958.

284. MILLER, A.: The in vitro binding of cobalt[60] labeled vitamin B_{12} by normal and leukemic sera. J. Clin. Invest. *37:*556, 1958.

284a. MILLER, A., AND SULLIVAN, J. F.: Some physicicochemical properties of the vitamin B_{12} binding substances of normal and chronic myelogenous leukemic sera. J. Lab. & Clin. Med. *53:*607, 1959.

285. HORRIGAN, D. L., AND HEINLE, R. W.: Refractory macrocytic anemia with defect in vitamin B_{12} binding and with response to normal plasma. J. Lab. & Clin. Med. *40:*811, 1952.

286. BETHELL, F. H.: Pteroylglutamic acid. XI (B). Requirements of man. *In* Sebrell, W. H., and Harris, R. S.: The Vitamins. New York, Academic Press, 1954, vol. 3.

287. WITTS, L. J.: Recent work on B vitamins in the blood and gastrointestinal tract, especially in relation to human diseases. Brit. M. Bull. *12:*14, 1956.

288. CHANARIN, J.: Blood folic acid. Brit. M. J. *1:*1179, 1958.

289. USDIN, E., PHILLIPS, P. N., AND TOENNIES, G.: Multiplicity of the folic acid-active factors of blood. J. Biol. Chem. *221:*865, 1956.

290. DENKO, C. W., GRUNDY, W. E., WHEELER, N. C., HENDERSON, C. R., FRIEDE-MANN, T. E., AND YOUMANS, J. B.: The excretion of B-complex vitamins by normal adults on a restricted intake. Arch. Biochem. *11:*109, 1946.

291. BLANCK, F. C.: Handbook of Food and Agriculture. New York, Reinhold, 1955.

292. TOEPFER, E. W., ZOOK, E. G., ORR, M. L., AND RICHARDSON, L. R.: Agriculture Handbook 29. United States Department of Agriculture, 1951.

293. SCHWEIGERT, B. S., POLLARD, A. E., AND ELVEHJEM, C. A.: The folic acid content of meats and the retention of this vitamin during cooking. Arch. Biochem. *10:*107, 1946.

294. IVES, M., POLLARD, A. E., ELVEHJEM, C. A., AND STRONG, F. M.: The nutritive value of canned foods. XVII. Pyridoxine, biotin, and "folic acid." J. Nutrition. *31:*347, 1946.

295. STOKSTAD, E. L. R.: Pteroylglutamic acid. VIII. Occurrence in foods. *In* Sebrell, W. H., Jr., and Harris, R. S.: The Vitamins. New York, Academic Press, 1954, vol. 3.

296. COLLINS, R. A., HARPER, A. E. SCHREIBER, M., AND ELVEHJEM, C. A.: The folic acid content and vitamin B_{12} content of the milk of various species. J. Nutrition. *43:*313, 1951.

297. ZUELZER, W. W.: Folic acid therapy in the anemias of infancy and childhood. J.A.M.A. *131:*7, 1946.

298. ——, AND OGDEN, F. N.: Megaloblastic anemia in infancy; a common syndrome responding specifically to folic acid therapy. A.M.A. Am. J. Dis. Child. *71:*211, 1946.

299. LUHBY, A. L., AND WHEELER, W. E.: Megaloblastic anemia of infancy. II. Failure of response to vitamin B_{12} and the metabolic role of folic acid and vitamin C. Ohio State University, Health Center J. *3:*1, 1949.

299a. ——: Megaloblastic anemia in infancy. III. Clinical considerations and analysis. J. Pediat. *54:*617, 1959.

300. GASSER, C.: Folsäure bei perniciosiformer Zeigenmilch-Anämie. Helvet. paediat. acta 3:301, 1948.

301. BRAESTRUP, P. W.: C-vitaminstudier hos spaedborn. Dissert. Copenhagen, Haase & Son, 1939.

302. MONTO, R. W., KAVANAUGH, D., AND REBUCK, J. W.: Severe nutritional macrocytic anemia in emotionally disturbed patients. Am. J. Clin. Nutrition. 6:105, 1958.

303. WALT, F., HOLMAN, S., AND HENDRICKSE, R. G.: Megaloblastic anaemia of infancy in kwashiorkor and other disease. Brit. M. J. 1:1199, 1956.

304. CHANARIN, I., MOLLIN, D. L., AND ANDERSON, B. B.: Folic acid deficiency and the megaloblastic anaemias. Proc. Roy. Soc. Med. 51:757, 1958.

305. LIEN-KENG, K., AND ODANG, O.: Megaloblastic anemia in infancy and childhood in Djakarta. A.M.A. Am. J. Dis. Child. 97:209, 1959.

306. STURGEON, P., AND CARPENTER, G.: Megaloblastic anemia of infancy. Response to vitamin B_{12}. Blood 5:458, 1950.

307. GELIN, G., AND IBORRA, M.: Les Anémies Mégaloblastiques de l'Enfance et les Problèmes de la Mégaloblastose. Paris, Masson, 1955.

307a. GERBASI, M.: L'anemie megaloblastique du norrisson. Rev. port. pediat. e puer. 21:1, 1958.

308. BETHELL, F. H.: Pteroylglutamic acid. IX (C). Effects of deficiency in man. In Sebrell, W. H., and Harris, R. S.: The Vitamins. New York, Academic Press, 1954, vol. 3.

309. KOTHARI, B. V., AND BHENDE, Y. M.: Nutritional megaloblastic anaemia. Indian J. M. Res. 37:347, 1949.

310. UNGLEY, C. C.: The pathogenesis of megaloblastic anaemias and the value of vitamin B_{12}. Brit. J. Nutrition. 6:299, 1952.

311. GIRDWOOD, R. H.: Some aspects of disordered folic acid metabolism in man. In Wolstenholme, G. E. W., and Cameron, M. P.: Ciba Foundation Symposium on Chemistry and Biology of Pteridines. London, J. & A. Churchill, 1954.

312. CHANARIN, I., ANDERSON, B. B., AND MOLLIN, D. L.: The absorption of folic acid. Brit. J. Haemat. 4:156, 1958.

313. COHEN, I.: Post-partum megaloblastic anemia. South African M. J. 27:627, 1953.

313a. LOWENSTEIN, L.: Vitamin B_{12} in pregnancy and the puerperium. Am. J. Clin. Nutrition. (in press).

314. BERRY, C. G.: Anaemia of pregnancy in Africans of Lagos. Brit. M. J. 2:819, 1955.

315. CHAUDHURI, S.: Vitamin B_{12} in megaloblastic anaemia of pregnancy and tropical nutritional macrocytic anaemia. Brit. M. J. 2:825, 1951.

316. PATEL, J. C., AND KOCHER, B. R.: Vitamin B_{12} in macrocytic anemia of pregnancy and the puerperium. Brit. M. J. 1:924, 1950.

317. VAN BUCHEM, F. S. P., AND NIEWIG, H. O.: Anaemia in pregnancy. Lancet 1:153, 1959.

318. VILTER, R. W.: Treatment of macrocytic anemia. Arch. Int. Med. 95:482, 1955.

319. MOORE, H. C., LILLIE, E. W., AND GATENBY, P. B. B.: The response of megaloblastic anemia of pregnancy to vitamin B_{12}. Irish J. M. S. 6:106, 1955.

320. KILLANDER, A.: Megaloblastic anemia associated with pregnancy or puerperium: Report of three cases with normal serum vitamin B_{12} levels and
subsequent response to treatment with vitamin B_{12}. Acta haemat. 19:9,
1958.

321. SCOTT, J. M.: Therapy in the megaloblastic anemias of pregnancy. Obst. &
Gynec. Surv. 10:370, 1955.

322. MOORE, C. V., VILTER, R., MINNICH, V., AND SPIES, T. D.: Nutritional macrocytic anemia in patients with pellagra or deficiency of the vitamin B
complex. J. Lab. & Clin. Med. 29:1226, 1944.

323. FOY, H., AND KONDI, A.: Treatment of megaloblastic anaemias. Relation of
penicillin to vitamin B_{12}. Lancet 2:360, 1953.

324. ADAMS, E. B.: Treatment of megaloblastic anaemia of pregnancy and the
puerperium with vitamin B_{12}. Brit. M. J. 2:398, 1956.

325. VILTER, C. F., SPIES, T. D., AND KOCH, M. B.: Further studies on folic acid
in the treatment of macrocytic anemia. South. M. J. 38:781, 1945.

326. GOODALL, J. W. O., GOODALL, H. I., AND BANNERJEE, D.: Folic acid in nutritional anaemia. Lancet 1:20, 1948.

327. RAMALINGASWAMI, V., AND MENON, P. S.: Folic acid in nutritional macrocytic anaemia. Indian J. M. Res. 37:471, 1949.

328. SPIES, T. D., DREIZEN, S., PARKER, G. S., AND SILBERMAN, D. J.: Detection
and treatment of nutritive failure in children. Recent observations.
J.A.M.A. 148:1376, 1952.

329. TASKER, P. W. G.: Correlation of serum vitamin B_{12} levels and urinary folic
acid in nutritional megaloblastic anaemia. Lancet 2:61, 1955.

330. DAS GUPTA, C. R., CHATTERJEA, J. B., GHOSH, S. K., AND BANNERJEE, D. K.:
Vitamin B_{12} concentration of serum in nutritional megaloblastic anaemia.
Bull. Calcutta Sch. Trop. Med. 3:101, 1956.

330a. RUBIN, C. E., BRANDBORG, L. L., PHELPS, P. C., AND TAYLOR, H. C., JR.: Studies
of celiac disease: I. The apparent identical and specific nature of the
duodenal and proximal jejunal lesion in celiac disease and idiopathic sprue.
Gastroenterology. To be published.

331. SPIES, T. D., SUAREZ, R. M., SUAREZ, R. M., JR., AND MORALES-HERNANDEZ, F.:
The therapeutic effect of folic acid in tropical sprue. Science 104:75, 1946.

332. DARBY, W. J., JONES, E., AND JOHNSON, H. C.: The use of synthetic L. casei
factor in the treatment of sprue. Science 103:108, 1946.

333. SPIES, T. D., LOPEZ, G. G., MENENDEZ, A., MINNICH, V., AND KOCH, M.: The
effect of folic acid on sprue. South. M. J. 39:30, 1946.

334. MANSON-BAHR, P. E. C., AND CLARKE, O.: Folic acid in tropical sprue. Lancet
2:903, 1946.

335. MORRISON, R. J. G., AND ST. JOHNSON, C. R.: Treatment of tropical sprue with
folic acid. Lancet 1:636, 1947.

336. GIRDWOOD, R. H.: A folic acid excretion test in the investigation of intestinal
malabsorption. Lancet 265:53, 1953.

337. ANDERSON, D. H., AND DI SANT'AGNESE, P. A.: The celiac syndrome. In
McQuarrie, I., and Kelley, V. C., Eds.: Brenneman's Practice of Pediatrics.
Hagerstown, Md., W. F. Prior, 1953, vol. 1, chap. 29.

338. Di Sant'Agnese, P. A.: Idiopathic celiac disease. II. Course and prognosis. Pediatrics 11:224, 1953.

339. Thompson, L.: Folic acid therapy in coeliac disease. Brit. M. J. 1:297, 1948.

340. Israels, M. C. G., and Sharp, J.: Idiopathic steatorrhea (non-tropical sprue) with megaloblastic anemia. Lancet 1:752, 1950.

341. Favorite, G. O.: The treatment of macrocytic anemia with synthetic L. casei factor (folic acid); a case report. Pennsylvania M. J. 49:855, 1946.

342. Zumoff, B.: Possible relationship of folic acid to uric acid metabolism as exemplified by a case of non-tropical sprue. Am. J. M. Sc. 225:674, 1953.

343. Cohen, B. S., Meyer, L. M., and Fadem, R.: Sprue refractory to vitamin B_{12}; satisfactory response to folic acid. Ann. Int. Med. 36:1533, 1952.

344. Davidson, L. S. P.: Pteroylglutamic acid (folic acid). Therapeutic indications and limitations. Edinburgh M. J. 55:400, 1948.

345. ——, Girdwood, R. H., and Innes, E. M.: Folic acid in the treatment of the sprue syndrome. Lancet 2:511, 1947.

346. Fox, H. J.: A comparison of pteroylglutamic acid and liver extract maintenance therapy in sprue. New England J. Med. 240:801, 1949.

347. Weir, J. F., and Comfort, M. W.: Folic acid therapy in non-tropical sprue: Results of treatment in seven cases. J. Lab. & Clin. Med. 32:1231, 1947.

348. Adlersberg, D., and Schein, J.: Clinical and pathologic studies in sprue. J.A.M.A. 134:1459, 1947.

349. Thiersch, J. B., and Philips, F. S.: Effects of 4-amino-pteroylglutamic acid in dogs with special reference to megaloblastosis. Proc. Soc. Exper. Biol. & Med. 71:484, 1949.

350. Nichol, C. A., and Welch, A. D.: On the mechanism of action of Aminopterin. Proc. Soc. Exper. Biol. & Med. 74:403, 1950.

351. Broquist, H. P., Stokstad, E. L. R., and Jukes, T. H.: Some biological and chemical properties of the citrovorum factor. J. Biol. Chem. 185:399, 1950.

352. Badenoch, J.: The use of labelled vitamin B_{12} and gastric biopsy in the investigation of anaemia. Proc. Roy. Soc. Med. 47:426, 1952.

353. Hawkins, C. F., and Meynell, M. J.: Macrocytosis and macrocytic anemia caused by anticonvulsant drugs. Quart. J. Med. 27:45, 1958.

354. Berlyne, N., Levine, M., and McGlashen, A.: Megaloblastic anemia following anticonvulsants. Brit. M. J. 1:1247, 1955.

355. Chalmers, J. N. M., and Boheimer, K.: Megaloblastic anemia and anticonvulsant therapy. Lancet 2:920, 1954.

356. Hawkins, C. F., and Meynell, M. J.: Megaloblastic anemia due to phenytoin sodium. Lancet 2:737, 1954.

357. Rhind, E. G., and Varadi, S.: Megaloblastic anemia due to phenytoin sodium. Lancet 2:921, 1954.

358. Fuld, H.: Megaloblastic anaemia following anticonvulsants. Brit. M. J. 1:1475, 1955.

359. Girdwood, R. H., and Lenman, J. A. R.: Megaloblastic anaemia occurring during primidone therapy. Brit. M. J. 1:146, 1956.

360. Newman, M. J. D., and Sumner, D. W.: Megaloblastic anemia following the use of primidone. Blood 12:183, 1957.

361. CALVERT, R. J., HURWORTH, E., AND MACBEAN, A. L.: Megaloblastic anemia from methophenobarbital. Blood *13*:894, 1958.

362. HOBSON, Q. J. G., SELWYN, J. G., AND MOLLIN, D. L.: Megaloblastic anaemia due to barbiturates. Lancet *271*:1079, 1956.

363. CHRISTENSON, W. N., ULTMANN, J. E., AND ROSEMAN, D. M.: Megaloblastic anemia during primidone (mysoline) therapy. J.A.M.A. *163*:940, 1957.

364. WEBSTER, J. M.: Megaloblastic anaemia due to phenytoin sodium. Lancet *2*:1017, 1954.

365. CHANARIN, I., ELMES, P. C., AND MOLLIN, D. L.: Folic-acid studies in megaloblastic anaemia due to primidone. Brit. M. J. *2*:80, 1958.

366. FALCO, E. A., GOODWIN, L. G., HITCHINGS, G. H., ROLLO, I. M., AND RUSSELL, P. B.: 2,4-diaminopyrimidines-a new series of antimalarials. Brit. J. Pharmacol. *6*:185, 1951.

367. MYATT, A. V., HERNANDEZ, T., AND COATNEY, G. R.: Studies in human malaria. XXXIII. The toxicity of pyrimethamine (daraprim) in man. Am. J. Trop. Med. *2*:788, 1953.

368. TAPIE, J., LAPORTE, J., MONNIER, J., RIBET, A., BERNADET, AND DAVÈRE: Anémie avec mégaloblastose médullaire au cours d'un traitement par la pyriméthamine (malocide). Bull. et mém. Soc. méd. hôp. Paris *74*:902, 1958.

369. HITCHINGS, G. H., ELION, G. B., AND SINGER, S.: Derivatives of condensed pyrimidine systems as antimetabolites. *In* Wolstenholme, G. E. M., and Cameron, M. P.: Ciba Foundation Symposium on Chemistry and Biology of Pteridines. Boston, Little, Brown & Co., 1954.

370. ——: Daraprim as an antagonist of folic and folinic acid. Tr. Roy. Soc. Trop. Med. & Hyg. *46*:467, 1952.

371. WOOLLEY, D. W.: Antimetabolites. Science *129*:615, 1959.

372. SPRAY, G. H., AND WITTS, L. J.: Results of three years' experience with microbiologic assay of vitamin B_{12} in serum. Brit. M. J. *1*:295, 1958.

373. NICHOL, G. A., AND WELCH, A. D.: Synthesis of citrovorum factor from folic acid by liver slices; augmentation by ascorbic acid. Proc. Soc. Exper. Biol. & Med. *74*:52, 1950.

374. BROQUIST, H. P., STOKSTAD, E. L. R., AND JUKES, T. H.: Biochemical studies with the "citrovorum factor." J. Lab. & Clin. Med. *38*:95, 1951.

375. MCMILLAN, R. B., AND INGLIS, J. C.: Scurvy: a survey of fifty-three cases. Brit. M. J. *2*:233, 1944.

376. BRONTE-STEWART, B.: The anaemia of adult scurvy. Quart. J. Med. *22*:309, 1953.

377. BROWN, A.: Megaloblastic anaemia associated with adult scurvy: report of a case which responded to synthetic ascorbic acid alone. Brit. J. Haemat. *1*:345, 1955.

378. ——: The anaemia of scurvy. Glasgow M. J. *32*:95, 1951.

379. METTIER, S. R., MINOT, G. R., AND TOWNSEND, W. C.: Scurvy in adults, especially the effect of food rich in vitamin C on blood formation. J.A.M.A. *95*:1089, 1930.

380. CRANDON, J. H., LUND, C. C., AND DILL, D. B.: Experimental human scurvy. New England J. Med. 223:353, 1940.

381. KREBS, H. A., PETERS, R. A., COWARD, K. H., MAPSON, L. W., PARSONS, L. G., PLATT, B. S., SPENCE, J. C., AND O'BRIEN, J. R. P.: Vitamin-C requirement of human adults. Experimental study of vitamin-C deprivation in man. Lancet 1:853, 1948.

382. ALDRICH, R. A., AND NELSON, E. N.: Megaloblastic anemia in infants. J.-Lancet 67:399, 1947.

383. MAY, C. D., NELSON, E. N., LOWE, C. U., AND SALMON, R. J.: Pathogenesis of megaloblastic anemia in infancy; interrelationship between pteroylglutamic acid and ascorbic acid. A.M.A. Am. J. Dis. Child. 80:191, 1950.

384. DAVIS, L. J., AND BROWN, A.: The Megaloblastic Anaemias. Springfield, Ill., Charles C Thomas, 1953.

385. EHRLICH, P., AND LAZARUS, A.: Histology of the Blood. Cambridge, University Press, 1900.

386. VAUGHN, J. M.: Leuco-erythroblastic anemia. J. Path. & Bact. 42:541, 1936.

387. WILSON, T. E.: Bone marrow in anemia. M. J. Australia 1:513, 1942.

388. BAEZ-VILLASENOR, J., AND SANCHEZ-MEDAL, L.: Case report: a case of erythemic myelosis (Di Guglielmo). Blood 8:1137, 1953.

389. DAMESHEK, W., AND GUNZ, F.: Leukemia. New York, Grune & Stratton, 1958.

390. BALDINI, M., FUDENBERG, H., FUKUTAKE, K., AND DAMESHEK, W.: The anemia of the Di Guglielmo symdrome. Blood 14:334, 1959.

391. PARAL, A.: Liver-resistant pernicious anemia with megaloblastosis of bone marrow terminating in acute leukemia. Rev. hémat. 4:655, 1949.

392. SINN, C. M., AND DICK, F. W.: Monocytic leukemia. Am. J. Med. 20:588, 1956.

393. ISRAELS, M. C. G.: Hemoglobinization of erythroblasts. J. Path. & Bact. 52:361, 1941.

394. LAMBIN, P., AND DE WEERDT, W.: Le probleme des megaloblastes. Rev. belge sc. méd. 10:282, 1938.

395. STONE, F. H.: Megaloblastic erythropoiesis in a case of myeloid leukemia during treatment. Glasgow M. J. 31:125, 1950.

396. DAMESHEK, W., AND BALDINI, M.: The Di Guglielmo syndrome. Blood 13:192, 1958.

397. WASSERMAN, L. R.: Personal communication, supported by slides of peripheral blood and bone marrow morphology.

398. ISRAELS, M. C. G., AND WILKINSON, J. F.: Achrestic anaemia. Quart. J. Med. 9:163, 1940.

399. DAVIDSON, L. S. P.: Refractory megaloblastic anemia. Blood 3:107, 1948.

400. DACIE, J. V., SMITH, M. D., WHITE, J. C., AND MOLLIN, D. L.: Refractory normoblastic anaemia: a clinical and haematological study of seven cases. Brit. J. Haemat. 5:56, 1959.

401. ROELSON, E., AND OHLSEN, A. S.: Achrestic anemia: completely refractory megaloblastic anemia. A case followed for nearly four years. Acta med. scandinav. 150:17, 1954.

401a. VILTER, R. W., AND MUELLER, J. F.: The growth and maturation of the erythrocyte. *In* BEAN, W. B., ED.: Monographs in Medicine, Series I. Baltimore, Williams and Wilkins, 1952.

401b. HUGULEY, C. M., JR., BAIN, J. A., RIVERS, S. L., AND SCOGGINS, R. B.: Refractory megaloblastic anemia associated with excretion of orotic acid. Blood *14*:615, 1959.

402. WATSON, C. J.: Macrocytic anemia. Illinois M. J. *82*:195, 1942.

403. DAMESHEK, W., AND INGALL, M.: Agranulocytosis (malignant neutropenia); report of 9 cases, 2 with recovery. Am. J. M. Sc. *181*:502, 1931.

404. CONLEY, C. L., GREEN, T. W., HARTMAN, R. C., AND KREVANS, J. R.: Prolonged treatment of pernicious anemia with vitamin B_{12}. Am. J. Med. *13*:284, 1952.

405. TEMPKA, T., AND BRAUN, B.: Mechanism of increased hemolysis in pernicious anemia and autohemolytic action of liver. Diet. Folia haemat. *48*:355, 1932.

405a. CHEVALLIER, P., BERNARD, J., BILSKI-PASQUIER, G., AND CHRISTOL, D.: La tuberculose aigue pseudoleucosique. Sémaine Hop. Paris. *30*:774, 1954.

406. KASSIRSKY, I. A.: Die Punktion des Knochenmarkes und die Blutbildung bei der visceralen Kinderleishmaniose. Diet. Folia haemat. *51*:352, 1934.

407. ROHR, K.: Knochensmarksmorphologie des Menschlichen Sternalpunktäts. Berlin, Urban & Schwartzenberg, 1937.

408. KOSZEWSKI, B. J.: The occurrence of megaloblastic erythropoiesis in patients with hemochromatosis. Blood 7:1182, 1952.

409. GILLMAN, T.: Cell enzymes and iron metabolism in anemias and siderosis. Nutrit. Rev. *16*:353, 1958.

410. GRUELUND, S.: Megaloblastic hemolytic anemia. Acta med. scandinav. (suppl. 239) *138*:101, 1950.

411. DEMURO, P., AND LEONARDI, G.: Hemopathic mediterranean syndrome. Acta med. scandinav. *138*:362, 1950.

412. GERIOLA, F.: Hemolytic splenomegaly associated with perniciosiform anemia. Inform. Med. Genova *3*:77, 1949.

413. JANDL, J. H., AND GREENBERG, M. S.: Bone-marrow failure due to relative nutritional deficiency in Cooley's hemolytic anemia. New England J. Med. *260*:461, 1959.

413a. JOHNSON, U., ROATH, O. S., AND KIRKPATRICK, C. I. F.: Nutritional megaloblastic anemia associated with sickle cell states. Blood *14*:535, 1959.

414. GRANVILLE, N., AND DAMESHEK, W.: Hemochromatosis with megaloblastic anemia responding to folic acid. New England J. Med. *258*:586, 1958.

415. MAIER, C.: Megaloblastic vitamin B_6 deficiency anemia with hemochromatosis. Schweiz. med. Wchnschr. *87*:1234, 1957.

416. CASTLE, W. B.: Commentary. *In* Beeson, P. B., Muschenheim, C., Castle, W. B., Harrison, T. R., Ingelfinger, F., and Bondy, P. K.: The Yearbook of Medicine, 1958–1959 Series. Chicago, The Year Book Publishers, 1958.

417. MOHLER, D. N., AND LEAVELL, B. S.: Aplastic anemia: an analysis of 50 cases. Ann. Int. Med. *49*:326, 1958.

418. MUELLER, J. F., AND WILL, J. J.: Interrelationship of folic acid, vitamin B_{12} and ascorbic acid in patients with megaloblastic anemia. Am. J. Clin. Nutrition. *3*:30, 1955.

418a. ARROWSMITH, W. R., BURRIS, M. B., AND SEGALOFF, A.: Production of megaloblastic marrow by administration of cortisone in aplastic anemia, with subsequent response to vitamin B_{12}; relationship not previously described. J. Lab. & Clin. Med. *42*:778, 1953.

419. CUSTER, R. P.: An Atlas of the Blood and Bone Marrow. Philadelphia, Saunders, 1949.

419a. WEISSBACH, H., TOOHEY, J., AND BARKER, H. A.: Isolation and properties of B_{12} coenzymes containing benzimidazole or dimethylbenzimidazole. Proc. Nat. Acad. Sc. *45*:521, 1959.

420. RICHMOND, J., AND DAVIDSON, S.: Subacute combined degeneration of the spinal cord in non-addisonian megaloblastic anaemia. Quart. J. Med. *27*:517, 1958.

421. SUAREZ, R. M.: Sprue. *In* Cecil, R. L., and Loeb, R. F.: A Textbook of Medicine, ed. 9. Philadelphia, W. B. Saunders, 1955.

422. NIEWIG, H. O., VAN BUCHEM, F. S. P., AND KROESE, W. F.: Vitamin B_{12} and pteroylglutamic acid in the treatment of megaloblastic anemias. Acta med. scandinav. *142*:45, 1952.

423. ——, FABER, J. G., DE VRIES, J. A., AND KROESE, W. F. S.: The relationship of vitamin B_{12} and folic acid in megaloblastic anemias. J. Lab. & Clin. Med. *44*:118, 1954.

424. BODIAN, D.: Nucleic acid in nerve cell regeneration. Symp. Soc. Exper. Biol. *1*:163, 1947.

425. ALEXANDER, W. F.: Pathomorphology of the nervous system in vitamin B_{12} deficiency. *In* Heinrich, H. C.: Vitamin B_{12} und Intrinsic Factor. Stuttgart, Ferdinand Enke, 1957.

426. ZIRM, K. L.: Uber die spezifische Anreicherung von Kobaltchlorophyllin im Nervensystem, ihre therapeutische Bedeutung und Beziehung zum Vitamin B_{12}. *In* Heinrich, H. C.: Vitamin B_{12} und Intrinsic Factor. Stuttgart, Ferdinand Enke, 1957.

427. CASPERSSON, T. O.: Cell Growth and Cell Function. New York, W. W. Norton, 1950.

428. STERN, J. R., TAYLOR, M. W., AND RUSSEL, W. C.: Relation of vitamin B_{12} to liver basophilia. Proc. Soc. Exper. Biol. & Med. *70*:551, 1949.

429. BAUER, H., AND HEINRICH, H. C.: Pathophysiologische Voraussetzungen zur therapeutischen Anwendung des Vitamin B_{12} bei neurologischen Erkrankungen. *In* Heinrich, H. C.: Vitamin B_{12} und Intrinsic Factor. Stuttgart, Ferdinand Enke, 1957.

430. PRUSOFF, W. H., TEPLY, L. J., AND KING, C. G.: The influence of pteroylglutamic acid on nucleic acid synthesis in Lactobacillus casei. J. Biol. Chem. *176*:1309, 1948.

431. HODSON, A. Z.: Compounds with "folic acid" activity. Arch. Biochem. *21*:330, 1949.

432. WAGLE, S. R., MEHTA, R., AND JOHNSON, B. C.: Vitamin B_{12} and protein biosynthesis. VI. Relation of vitamin B_{12} to amino acid activation. J. Biol. Chem. *233*:619, 1958.

433. NEILL, D. W., AND WEAVER, J. A.: Amino acid and protein metabolism in pernicious anemia. Brit. J. Haemat. 4:447, 1958.

434. FRASER, M. J., AND HOLDSWORTH, E. S.: Vitamin B_{12} and protein biosynthesis in chick liver. Nature 1:519, 1959.

435. ARNSTEIN, H. R. V., AND SIMKIN, J. L.: Vitamin B_{12} and protein biosynthesis in rat liver. Nature 1:523, 1959.

436. NEILL, D. W., AND WEAVER, J. A.: A study of some metabolic processes dependent on coenzyme "A" in pernicious anemia. Acta haemat. 21:23, 1959.

437. SMITHBURN, K. C., AND ZERFAS, L. G.: The neural symptoms and signs in pernicious anemia. Arch. Neurol. & Psychiat. 25:1110, 1931.

438. HYLAND, H. H. WATTS, G. O., AND FARQUHARSON, R. F.: Course of subacute combined degeneration of spinal cord. Canad. M. A. J. 65:295, 1951.

439. DAVIDSON, S.: Clinical picture of pernicious anemia prior to introduction of liver therapy in 1926 and in Edinburgh subsequent to 1944. Brit. M. J. 1:241, 1957.

440. GREENFIELD, J. G., AND CARMICHAEL, E. A.: The peripheral nerves in cases of subacute combined degeneration of the cord. Brain 58:483, 1935.

441. VAN DER SCHEER, W. M., AND KOEK, H. C.: Peripheral nerve lesions in cases of pernicious anemia. Acta psychiat. et neurol. 13:61, 1938.

442. JEWESBURY, E. C. C.: Subacute combined degeneration of the cord and achlorhydric peripheral neuropathies without anaemia. Lancet 2:307, 1954.

443. CASTLE, W. B.: The anemias. In Cecil, R. L., and Loeb, R. F.: A Textbook of Medicine, ed. 10. Philadelphia, W. B. Saunders, 1959.

444. UNGLEY, C. C.: Treatment with vitamin B_{12} in haematological disorders. In Heinrich, H. C.: Vitamin B_{12} and Intrinsic Factor. Stuttgart, Ferdinand Enke, 1957.

445. HEATON, J. M., McCORMICK, A. J. A., AND FREEMAN, A. G.: Tobacco amblyopia: a clinical manifestation of vitamin-B_{12} deficiency. Lancet 2:286, 1958.

446. HAMILTON, H. E., ELLIS, P. P., AND SHEETS, R. F.: Visual impairment due to optic neuropathy in pernicious anemia: report of a case and review of the literature. Blood 14:378, 1959.

446a. HARRIS, C. E. C.: Snares and delusions in the recognition of "pernicious anemia." Connecticut Med. J. 12:543, 1958.

447. VICTOR, M., AND LEAR, A. A.: Subacute combined degeneration of the spinal cord. Current concepts of the disease process. Value of serum vitamin B_{12} determinations in clarifying some of the common clinical problems. Am. J. Med. 20:896, 1956.

448. WOLTMAN, H. W., AND HECK, F. J.: Funicular degeneration of spinal cord without pernicious anemia: neurologic aspects of sprue, nontropical sprue and idiopathic steatorrhea. Arch. Int. Med. 60:292, 1937.

449. ARIAS, I. M., APT, L., AND POLLYCOVE, M.: Absorption of radioactive vitamin B_{12} in nonanemic patients with combined-system disease. New England J. Med. 253:1005, 1955.

450. ELLENBOGEN, L., WILLIAMS, W. L., RABINER, S. F., AND LICHTMAN, H. C.: An

improved urinary excretion test as an assay for intrinsic factor. Proc. Soc. Exper. Biol. & Med. 89:357, 1955.

451. SCHILLING, R. F.: Intrinsic factor studies. II. The effect of gastric juice on the urinary excretion of radioactivity after the oral administration of radioactive vitamin B12. J. Lab. & Clin. Med. 42:860, 1953.

452. Ross, G. I. M.: Vitamin B12 assay in body fluids using Euglena gracilis. J. Clin. Path. 5:250, 1952.

453. SPRAY, G. H.: An improved method for the rapid estimation of vitamin B12 in serum. Clin. Sc. 14:661, 1955.

454. BOSSAK, E. T., WANG, C. I., AND ADLERSBERG, D.: Clinical aspects of the malabsorption syndrome (idiopathic sprue). Observations in 94 patients. J. Mount Sinai Hosp. (New York) 24:286, 1957. Simultaneously published in Adlersberg, D.: The Malabsorption Syndrome. New York, Grune & Stratton, 1957.

455. BETHELL, F. H., AND HARRINGTON, B. D.: Incidence and significance of disease of gall bladder and liver in pernicious anemia. Am. J. Digest. Dis. & Nutrition. 1:256, 1934.

456. BROWN, M. R.: The pathology of the gastro-intestinal tract in pernicious anemia and subacute combined degeneration of the spinal cord. New England J. Med. 210:473, 1934.

457. BOYDEN, E. A., AND LAYNE, J. A.: The gall bladder in patients with pernicious anemia: a study of non-visualization and rate of emptying. Gastroenterology 4:121, 1945.

458. SINGER, K., KING, J. C., AND ROBIN, S.: The life span of the megalocyte and the hemolytic syndrome of pernicious anemia. J. Lab. & Clin. Med. 33:1068, 1948.

459. HAMILTON, H. E., DeGOWIN, E. L., SHEETS, R. F., JANNEY, C. D., AND ELLIS, J. A.: Studies with inagglutinable erythrocyte counts. VI. Accelerated destruction of normal adult erythrocytes in pernicious anemia; contribution of hemolysis to the oligocythemia. J. Clin. Invest. 33:191, 1954.

460. LONDON, I. M., AND WEST, R.: The formation of bile pigment in pernicious anemia. J. Biol. Chem. 184:359, 1950.

460a. POLLYCOVE, M.: Bone marrow hemolysis in anemia. J. Clin. Invest. 38:1031, 1959.

461. INGELFINGER, F. J.: Diseases of the gallbladder and bile ducts. In Harrison, T. R., Adams, R. D., Bennett, I. L., Jr., Resnik, W. H., Thorn, G. W., and Wintrobe, M. M.: Principles of Internal Medicine. New York, McGraw-Hill, 1958.

461a. WATSON, C. J.: Cholelithiasis. Cholecystitis. In CECIL, R. L., AND LOEB, R. F., EDS.: A Textbook of Medicine, tenth ed. Philadelphia, W. B. Saunders, 1959.

462. SCHILLING, R. F., AND HARRIS, J. W.: Liver function in untreated addisonian pernicious anemia. J. Lab. & Clin. Med. 40:718, 1952.

462a. TALBOTT, J. H.: Gout and blood dyscrasias. Medicine 38:173, 1959.

463. REIMANN, F.: Leberkrankung und perniziöse Anämie. In Heinrich, H. C.: Vitamin B12 und Intrinsic Factor. Stuttgart, Ferdinand Enke, 1957.

464. ——: Leberkrankung und perniziöse Anämie. Blut *4*:261, 1958.

465. STEVENSON, T. D., AND BEARD, M. F.: Serum vitamin B_{12} content in liver disease. New England J. Med. *260*:206, 1959.

465a. DE GRUCHY, G. C.: Clinical Haematology in Medical Practice. Springfield, Ill., C. C Thomas, 1958.

466. CAMERON, D. G., BENSLEY, E. H., AND WOOD, P.: Latent steatorrhea. Ann. Int. Med. *37*:553, 1952.

467. JUERGENS, J. L., SCHOLZ, D. A., AND WOLLAEGER, E. E.: Severe osteomalacia associated with occult steatorrhea due to non-tropical sprue. Arch. Int. Med. *98*:774, 1956.

468. STURGIS, C. C., AND ISAACS, R.: Pernicious anemia. *In* Downey, H.: Handbook of Hematology. New York, Paul B. Hoeber, 1938, vol. 3.

468a. MARSHALL, R. A., AND JANDL, J. H.: Diagnostic use of small doses of folic acid in megaloblastic anemias. Clinical Research *7*:206, 1959.

468b. MCKELLAR, M.: Investigation of megaloblastic anemias. New Zealand J. Med. *58*:18, 1959.

469. HAM, T. H.: A Syllabus of Laboratory Examinations in Clinical Diagnosis. Cambridge, Harvard University Press, 1952.

470. BLOOMFIELD, A. L., AND POLLARD, W. S.: Gastric Anacidity. New York, Macmillan, 1933.

471. SEGAL, H. L., MILLER, L. L., AND MORTON, J. J.: Determination of gastric acidity without intubation by use of cation exchange indicator compounds. Proc. Soc. Exper. Biol. & Med. *74*:218, 1950.

472. RECHTSCHAFFEN, J. S., VENET, L., AND WEINGARTEN, M.: Gastric acidity determination procedures. Comparison of a tubeless method with azure A resin compound and an intubation method with histamine. J.A.M.A. *164*: 1467, 1957.

473. BOLT, R. J., OSSIUS, T. G., AND POLLARD, H. M.: A clinical evaluation of tubeless gastric analysis. Gastroenterology. *32*:34, 1957.

474. DENBOROUGH, M. A., RETIEF, F. P., AND WITTS, L. J.: Tubeless gastric analysis. Brit. M. J. *1*:1213, 1958.

475. HERBERT, V.: Development of a possible in vitro assay for intrinsic factor. Proc. Soc. Exper. Biol. & Med. *97*:668, 1958.

476. ——, CASTRO, Z., AND WASSERMAN, L. R.: Rapid in vitro "assay" of intrinsic factor in human gastric juice. Clinical Research *7*:259, 1959.

477. GRÄSBECK, R.: Studies on the vitamin B_{12}-binding principle and other biocolloids of human gastric juice. Acta med. scandinav. suppl. 314, 1956.

478. BERTCHER, R. W., MEYER, L. M., AND MILLER, I. F.: Co^{60} vitamin B_{12} binding capacity of normal human saliva. Proc. Soc. Exper. Biol. & Med. *99*:513, 1958.

479. OKUDA, K., GRÄSBECK, R., AND CHOW, B. F.: Bile and vitamin B_{12} absorption. J. Lab. & Clin. Med. *51*:17, 1958.

480. GRÄSBECK, R., NYBERG, W., AND REIZENSTEIN, P.: Biliary and fecal vit. B_{12} excretion in man. An isotope study. Proc. Soc. Exper. Biol. & Med. *97*:780, 1958.

481. MILLER, O. N.: Studies on an interaction among serum protein, materials containing intrinsic factor and vitamin B_{12}. Arch. Biochem. 72:8, 1957.

482. ——, AND UNGLAUB, W. G.: A study of etiology of macrocytic anemia. J. Clin. Invest. 36:915, 1957.

483. HUTNER, S. H., CURY, A., AND BAKER, H.: Microbiological assays. Analyt. Chem. 30:849, 1958.

484. COATES, M. E., AND FORD, J. E.: Methods of measurement of vitamin B_{12}. Biochem. Soc. Symp. 13:36, 1955.

485. MOLLIN, D. L., AND ROSS, G. I. M.: The pathophysiology of vitamin B_{12} deficiency in the megaloblastic anaemias. In Heinrich, H. C.: Vitamin B_{12} und Intrinsic Factor. Stuttgart, Ferdinand Enke, 1957.

485a. LOWENSTEIN, L.: Personal communication.

486. SOBOTKA, H., BAKER, H., AND ZIFFER, H.: Vitamin B_{12} distribution between plasma and cells. Vitamin B_{12} Symposium, New York Medical College. April 11, 1958. Am. J. Clin. Nutrition. (in press).

487. HERBERT, V.: Discussion of reference 486. Am. J. Clin. Nutrition. (In press).

488. ——: Unpublished data.

489. ——, WASSERMAN, L. R., FRANK, O., PASHER, I., AND BAKER, H. (Intro. by SOBOTKA, H.): Value of fasting serum "folic acid" levels. Fed. Proc. 18:246, 1959.

489a. BAKER, H., HERBERT, V., FRANK, O., PASHER, I., WASSERMAN, L. R., AND SOBOTKA, H.: A microbiologic method for detecting folic acid deficiency in man. Clin. Chem. 5:275, 1959.

489b. HERBERT, V., BAKER, H., FRANK, O., PASHER, I., SOBOTKA, H., AND WASSERMAN, L. R.: The measurement of folic acid activity in serum: a diagnostic aid in the differentiation of the megaloblastic anemias. Blood (In press).

490. DENKO, C. W.: Pteroylglutamic acid clearance in normal adults. J. Appl. Physiol. 3:559, 1951.

491. SPRAY, G. H., AND WITTS, L. J.: The utilization of folic acid given by mouth. Clin. Sc. 11:273, 1952.

492. CLARK, S. L., JR.: Oral folic acid tolerance test in normal human subjects and patients with pernicious anemia. Proc. Soc. Exper. Biol. & Med. 82:25, 1953.

493. DENKO, C. W., GRUNDY, W. E., PORTER, J. W., BERRYMAN, G. H., FRIEDEMANN, T. E., AND YOUMANS, J. B.: The excretion of B-complex vitamins in the urine and feces of seven normal adults. Arch. Biochem. 10:33, 1946.

494. REGISTER, U. D., AND SARETT, H. P.: Urinary excretion of vitamin B_{12}, folic acid, and citrovorum factor in human subjects on various diets. Proc. Soc. Exper. Biol. & Med. 77:837, 1951.

495. SUAREZ, R. M., WELCH, A. D., HEINLE, R. W., SUAREZ, R. M., JR., AND NELSON, E. N.: Effectiveness of conjugated forms of folic acid in the treatment of tropical sprue. J. Lab. & Clin. Med. 31:1294, 1946.

496. SWENSEID, M. E., BIRD, O. D., BROWN, R. A., AND BETHELL, F. H.: Metabolic function of pteroylglutamic acid and its hexaglutamyl conjugate. J. Lab. & Clin. Med. 32:23, 1947.

497. CHANARIN, I., MOLLIN, D. L., AND ANDERSON, B. B.: The clearance from the

plasma of folic acid injected intravenously in normal subjects and patients with megaloblastic anaemia. Brit. J. Haemat. *4:*435, 1958.

498. COX, E. V., MEYNELL, M. J., COOKE, W. T., AND GADDIE, R.: The folic acid excretion test in the steatorrhea syndrome. Gastroenterology *35:*390, 1958.

499. BOREK, B. A., AND WAELSCH, H.: The enzymatic degradation of histidine. J. Biol. Chem. *205:*459, 1953.

500. TABOR, H., AND MEHLER, A. H.: Isolation of N-formyl-L-glutamic acid as an intermediate in the enzymatic degradation of L-histidin. J. Biol. Chem. *201:*559, 1954.

501. SILVERMAN, M., GARDINER, R. C., AND BAKERMAN, H. A.: The nature of glutamic acid excreted in folic acid deficiency. J. Biol. Chem. *194:*815, 1952.

502. TABOR, H., SILVERMAN, M., MEHLER, A. H., DAFT, F. S., AND BAUER, H.: L-histidine conversion to a urinary glutamic acid derivative in folic-deficient rats. J. Am. Chem. Soc. *75:*756, 1953.

503. DAFT, F. S.: Certain aspects of the relations between nutrition and liver function. *In* Brauer, R.: Liver Function. A Symposium on Approaches to the Quantitative Description of Liver Function. Publication #4. Washington, D. C., American Institute of Biological Sciences, 1958.

504. BROQUIST, H. P.: Evidence for the excretion of formiminoglutamic acid following folic acid antagonist therapy in acute leukemia. J. Am. Chem. Soc. *78:*6205, 1956.

505. LUHBY, A. L.: Observations on the excretion of formiminoglutamic acid in folic acid deficiency in man. Clinical Research Proceedings *5:*8, 1957.

506. TABOR, H., AND WYNGARDEN, L.: A method for the determination of formiminoglutamic acid in urine. J. Clin. Invest. *37:*824, 1958.

507. HIATT, H. H., GOLDSTEIN, M., AND TABOR, H.: Urinary excretion of formiminoglutamic acid by human subjects after antifolic acid therapy. J. Clin. Invest. *37:*829, 1958.

508. LUHBY, A. L., COOPERMAN, J. M., TELLER, D. N., AND DONNENFELD, A. M.: Excretion of formiminoglutamic acid in folic acid deficiency states. J. Clin. Invest. *37:*915, 1958.

509. SILVERMAN, M., GARDINER, R. C., AND CONDIT, P. T.: A method for the detection of N-formiminoglutamic acid in urine. J. Nat. Cancer Inst. *20:*71, 1958.

510. BROQUIST, H. P., AND LUHBY, A. L.: Detection and isolation of formiminoglutamic acid from urine in folic acid deficiency in humans. Proc. Soc. Exper. Biol. & Med. *100:*349, 1959.

511. LUHBY, A. L., COOPERMAN, J. M., AND TELLER, D. N.: Urinary excretion of formiminoglutamic acid: Application in diagnosis of clinical folic acid deficiency. Am. J. Clin. Nutrition. *7:*397, 1959.

512. HERBERT, V., BAKER, H., FRANK, O., PASHER, I., WASSERMAN, L. R., AND SOBOTKA, H.: Unpublished data.

513. SILVERMAN, M., AND PITNEY, A. J.: Dietary methionine and the excretion of formiminoglutamic acid by the rat. J. Biol. Chem. *233:*1179, 1958.

514. RABINOWITZ, J., AND TABOR, H.: The urinary excretion of formic acid and formiminoglutamic acid in folic acid deficiency. J. Biol. Chem. 233:252, 1958.

514a. HIATT, H. H., RABINOWITZ, J. C., TOCH, R., AND GOLDSTEIN, M.: Effects of folic acid antagonist therapy on urinary excretion of formic acid by humans. Proc. Soc. Exper. Biol. & Med. 98:144, 1958.

515. HEINLE, R. W., WELCH, A. D., SCHARF, V., MEACHAM, G. C., AND PRUSOFF, W. H.: Studies of excretion (and absorption) of Co60-labeled vitamin B_{12} in pernicious anemia. Tr. A. Am. Physicians 65:214, 1952.

516. BOOTH, C. C., AND MOLLIN, D. L.: Plasma, tissue and urinary radioactivity after oral administration of 56Co-labelled B_{12}. In Heinrich, H. C.: Vitamin B_{12} und Intrinsic Factor. Stuttgart, Ferdinand Enke, 1957.

517. GLASS, G. B. J., BOYD, L. J., GELLIN, G. A., AND STEPHANSON, L.: Uptake of radioactive vitamin B_{12} by the liver in humans: test of measurement of intestinal absorption of vitamin B_{12} and intrinsic factor activity. Arch. Biochem. 51:251, 1954.

518. ELLENBOGEN, L., AND WILLIAMS, W. L.: Quantitative assay of intrinsic factor by urinary excretion of radioactive vitamin B_{12}. Blood 13:582, 1958.

519. REISNER, E. H., JR., ROSENBLUM, C., AND MORGAN, M. C.: Urinary excretion of orally administered Co60-vitamin B_{12} in normal subjects and patients with pernicious anemia sprue. Clincal Research Proceedings 2:56, 1954.

520. RATH, C. E., MCCURDY, P. R., SCHREINER, G. E., AND DUFFY, B. J.: The effect of renal disease on the urinary excretion of cobalt 60 vitamin B_{12}. In Proceedings of the Sixth International Congress of the International Society of Hematology. New York, Grune & Stratton, 1958.

521. DUNN, A. L., WALSH, J. R., AND HOLTHAUS, J. M.: Radioactive cyanocobalamin (vitamin B_{12}) in renal disease. Arch. Int. Med. 101:927, 1958.

522. ROSENBLUM, C., AND GETHARD, P.: Personal communication.

523. BUCHHOLZ, C. H.: Concentration of vitamin B_{12} from urine by adsorption on carbon. J. Lab. & Clin. Med. 52:653, 1958.

524. HAWKINS, C. F.: Value of serum iron levels in assessing effect of haematinics in the macrocytic anaemias. Brit. M. J. 1:383, 1955.

525. VILTER, R. W., HORRIGAN, D., MUELLER, J. F., JARROLD, T., VILTER, C. F., HAWKINS, V., AND SEAMAN, A.: Studies on the relationships of vitamin B_{12}, folic acid, thymine, uracil, and methyl group donors in persons with pernicious anemia and related megaloblastic anemias. Blood 5:695, 1950.

526. CONLEY, C. L., AND KREVANS, J. R.: Development of nuerologic manifestations of pernicious anemia during multivitamin therapy. New England J. Med. 245:529, 1951.

527. BERK, L., DENNY-BROWN, D., FINLAND, M., AND CASTLE, W. B.: Effectiveness of vitamin B_{12} in combined system disease. Rapid progression of neurologic manifestations and absence of allergic reactions in a patient sensitive to injectable liver extracts. New England J. Med. 239:328, 1948.

528. SCHIEVE, J. F., AND RUNDLES, R. W.: Response of lingual manifestations of

pernicious anemia to pteroylglutamic acid and vitamin B_{12}. J. Lab. & Clin. Med. *34*:439, 1949.

529. WOLFF, R.: La position du foie dans le métabolisme normal et pathologique de la vitamine B_{12}. *In* Heinrich, H. C.: Vitamin B_{12} und Intrinsic Factor. Stuttgart, Ferdinand Enke, 1957.

530. DARBY, W. J.: Folic acid and citrovorum factor in human nutrition. Nutrition Symp. Series, No. 7. New York, National Vitamin Foundation, Inc., 1953.

531. UNGLAUB, W. G., AND GOLDSMITH, G. A.: Folic acid and vitamin B_{12} in medical practice. J.A.M.A. *161*:623, 1956.

532. ROSS, J. F., BELDING, H., AND PAEGEL, B. L.: The development and progression of subacute combined degeneration of the spinal cord in patients with pernicious anemia treated with synthetic pteroylglutamic (folic) acid. Blood *3*:68, 1948.

533. WRIGHT, L. D., SKEGGS, H. R., AND HUFF, J. W.: The ability of thymidine to replace vitamin B_{12} as a growth factor for certain lactobacilli. J. Biol. Chem. *175*:475, 1948.

534. BOK, J., FABER, J. G., DE VRIES, W. F., KROESE, W. F. S., AND NIEWIG, H. O.: The effect of pteroylglutamic acid on the serum vitamin B_{12} concentration in pernicious anemia in relapse. J. Lab. & Clin. Med. *51*:667, 1958.

535. A.M.A. COUNCIL ON FOODS AND NUTRITION: Vitamin preparations as dietary supplements and as therapeutic agents. J.A.M.A. *169*:41, 1959.

536. MOORE, C. V.: Pernicious anemia. *In* Conn, H. F.: Current Therapy-1959. Philadelphia, W. B. Saunders, 1959.

537. HARRIS, J. W.: Aggravation of clinical manifestations of folic acid deficiency by small daily doses of vitamin B_{12}. Am. J. Med. *21*:461, 1956.

538. COX, E. V., MEYNELL, M. J., COOKE, W. T., AND GADDIE, R.: Folic acid and cyanocobalamin in pernicious anaemia. Clin. Sc. *17*:693, 1958.

539. NELSON, R. S., AND DOCTOR, V. M.: The vitamin B_{12} content of human liver as determined by bio-assay of needle biopsy material. Ann. Int. Med. *49*:1361, 1958.

540. GROSSOWICZ, N., HOCHMAN, A., ARONOVITCH, J., IZAK, G., AND RACHMILE-WITZ, M.: Malignant growth in the liver and serum vitamin B_{12} levels. Lancet *1*:1116, 1957.

541. CONLEY, C. L., KREVANS, J. R., CHOW, B. F., BURROWS, C., AND LANG, C. A.: Observations on the absorption, utilization and excretion of vitamin B_{12}. J. Lab. & Clin. Med. *38*:84, 1951.

542. CHESTERMAN, D. C., CUTHBERTSON, W. F. J., AND PEGLER, H. F.: Vitamin B_{12} excretion studies. Biochem. J. *48*:li, 1951.

543. REISNER, E. H., JR., AND WEINER, L.: The treatment of pernicious anemia with massive parenteral doses of vitamin B_{12}. Blood *8*:81, 1953.

544. SOKOLOFF, M. S., SANNEMAN, E. H., JR., AND BEARD, M. F.: Urinary excretion of vitamin B_{12}. Blood *7*:243, 1952.

545. MOLLIN, D. L., AND ROSS, G. I. M.: Vitamin B_{12} concentrations of serum and urine in the first 72 hours after intramuscular injection of the vitamin. J. Clin. Path. *6*:54, 1953.

546. Mollin, D. L., and Ross, G. I. M.: Serum vitamin B_{12} concentration of patients with megaloblastic anaemia after treatment with vitamin B_{12}, folic acid, or folinic acid. Brit. M. J. 2:640, 1953.

547. Unglaub, W. G., Miller, O. N., and Goldsmith, G. A.: "Saturation" studies with vitamin B_{12} in human subjects. Am. J. Clin. Nutrition 6:535, 1958.

548. Goodman, L. S., and Gilman, A.: The Pharmacological Basis of Therapeutics, ed. 2. New York, Macmillan, 1955.

549. Goldblatt, S.: On the intravenous administration of cyanocobalamin. Am. J. Clin. Nutrition. 3:129, 1955.

550. Chow, B. F.: Personal communication to reference 482.

551. Hall, B. E., Krusen, F. H., and Woltman, H. W.: Vitamin B_{12} and coordination exercises for combined degeneration of the spinal cord in pernicious anemia. J.A.M.A. 141:257, 1949.

552. Gräsbeck, R.: Maintenance treatment in pernicious anaemia. Lancet 1:206. 1959.

552a. Rundles, R. W.: Prognosis in neurologic manifestations of pernicious anemia. Blood 1:209, 1946.

552b. Bethell, F. H., and Sturgis, C.: The relation of therapy in pernicious anemia to changes in the nervous system. Blood 3:57, 1948.

553. O'Connor, J. S., Davis, R. L., Langworthy, O. R., and Chow, B. F.: Metabolic studies of vitamin B_{12} and Depinar in multiple sclerosis (MS) and clinically healthy subjects. Fed Proc. 17:528, 1958.

553a. Thompson, R. E., and Hecht, R. A.: Studies on a long-acting vitamin B_{12} preparation. Am. J. Clin. Nutrit. 7:311, 1959.

554. Hemsted, E. H., and Mills, J.: Vitamin B_{12} in pernicious anemia. Lancet 2:1302, 1958.

555. Nieburgs, H. E.: Cytologic technics for office and clinic. Postgrad. Med. 23:309, 1958.

556. Tanaka, K. R., and Clifford, G. O.: Spontaneous remission in pernicious anemia. Report of a case. New England J. Med. 258:7, 1958.

557. Glass, G. B. J.: Biochemistry and physiology of Castle's intrinsic factor and its relationship to the metabolism of vitamin B_{12}. Rev. hémat. 10:137, 1955.

558. Estren, S., and Wasserman, L. R.: Pernicious anemia. I. Remission by small oral doses of purified vitamin B_{12}. Proc. Soc. Exper. Biol. & Med. 91:499, 1956.

558a. Schwartz, S. O., Friedman, I. A., and Gant, H. L.: Long-term evaluation of vitamin B_{12} in treatment of pernicious anemia. J.A.M.A. 157:229, 1955.

559. Chalmers, J. N. M., and Shinton, N. K.: Absorption of orally administered vitamin B_{12} in pernicious anemia. Lancet 2:1298, 1958.

560. Brody, E. A., Estren, S., and Wasserman, L. R.: Treatment of pernicious anemia by oral administration of vitamin B_{12} without added intrinsic factor. New England J. Med. 260:361, 1959.

561. Conley, C. L., and Krevans, J. R.: New developments in the diagnosis and treatment of pernicious anemia. Ann. Int. Med. 43:758, 1955.

562. Reisner, E. H., Jr., Weiner, L., Schittone, M. T., and Henck, E. A.: Oral

treatment of pernicious anemia with vitamin B_{12} without intrinsic factor. New England J. Med. *253*:502, 1955.

563. MILLER, O. N., RANEY, J. L., AND HUNTER, F. M.: Effect of intrinsic factor on uptake of radioactive vitamin B_{12} by slices of rat liver. Fed. Proc. *16*:393, 1957.

564. ——, AND HUNTER, F. M.: Stimulation of vit. B_{12} uptake in tissue slices by intrinsic factor concentrate. Proc. Soc. Exper. Biol. & Med. *96*:39, 1957.

565. BASTROP-MADSEN, P., AND PAULSEN, L.: Oral treatment of megaloblastic anaemia with small amounts of vitamin B_{12} and intrinsic factor. Acta haemat. *13*:193, 1955.

566. SCHWARTZ, M., LOUS, P., AND MEULENGRACHT, E.: Reduced effect of heterologous intrinsic factor after prolonged oral treatment in pernicious anemia. Lancet *1*:751, 1957.

567. KRISTENSEN, O., LUND, J., OHLSEN, A. S., AND PEDERSON, J.: Maintenance therapy in pernicious anemia controlled by determining vitamin B_{12} level in plasma. Lancet *1*:1266, 1957.

568. LOWENSTEIN, L., BRUNTON, L., SHAPIRO, L., DE LEEUW, N., AND DUFRESNE, M.: Maintenance therapy of pernicious anaemia with oral administration of intrinsic factor and vitamin B_{12}. Canad. M. A. J. *77*:923, 1957.

569. BERLIN, R., BERLIN, H., BRANTE, G., AND SJOBERG, S.-G.: Failures in long-term treatment of pernicious anemia with B_{12}-intrinsic factor preparations. Acta med. scandinav. *161*:143, 1958.

570. SCHWARTZ, M., LOUS, P., AND MEULENGRACHT, E.: Absorption of vitamin B_{12} in pernicious anemia. Defective absorption induced by prolonged oral treatment. Lancet *2*:1200, 1958.

571. STOKES, J. B., AND PITNEY, W. R.: Pernicious anaemia treated orally with "Bifacton." Refractoriness to potent animal intrinsic factor. Brit. M. J. *1*:322, 1958.

572. LICHTMAN, H. C., ELLENBOGEN, L., AND WILLIAMS, W. L.: Absorption of vitamin B_{12} by pernicious anemia patients before and after maintenance on an intrinsic factor concentrate. Third Vitamin B_{12} Symposium, New York Academy of Medicine. (Jan. 31–Feb. 1) 1958. See also: WILLIAMS, W. L.: Absorption of vitamin B_{12} via intrinsic factor concentrate. Fed. Proc. *18*:351, 1959.

573. FOUTS, P. J., HELMER, O. M., AND CHERNISH, S. M.: Absorption of radioactive B_{12} in patients with pernicious anemia after long term oral and parenteral therapy. The American College of Physicians, Fortieth Annual Session, Chicago, (April 20–24) 1959.

574. BERLIN, R., BERLIN, H., BRANTE, G., AND SJOBERG, S.-G.: Refractoriness to intrinsic factor-B_{12} preparations abolished by massive doses of intrinsic factor. Acta med. scandinav. *162*:317, 1958.

575. SCHWARTZ, M.: Intrinsic-factor-inhibiting substance in serum of orally treated patients with pernicious anemia. Lancet *2*:61, 1958.

576. TAYLOR, K. B., AND MORTON, J. A.: An antibody to Castle's intrinsic factor. Lancet *1*:29, 1958.

577. HERBERT, V.: Unpublished data.

578. GYORGY, P., TOCANTINS, L. M., MILLER, F. R., AND WEISS, A.: Hematopoiesis, blood group substance, and bifidus factor. Tr. A. Am. Physicians. *67*:117, 1954.

579. LATNER, A. L., MERRILLS, R. J., AND RAINE, L. C. D. P.: Further observations on the isolation and chemical composition of Castle's intrinsic factor. Biochem. J. *57*:xix, 1954.

580. SPRINGER, G. F.: Uber fucosehaltige Mucine vorweigend entodermalen Ursprungs mit Blutgruppen- und anderen biologischen Eigenschaften. Klin. Wchnschr. *33*:347, 1955.

581. VAN BAAL, J. P. W., WIJMENGA, H. G., AND VAN DER HART, M.: Blood group substance activity of intrinsic factor preparations. Biochim. et biophys. acta *17*:600, 1955.

581a. TAYLOR, K. B., AND MORTON, J. A.: An antibody to Castle's intrinsic factor. J. Path. & Bact. *77*:117, 1959.

581b. LOWENSTEIN, L., COOPER, B. A., BRUNTON, L., AND GARTHA, S.: Antibodies in human and rabbit sera to hog intrinsic factor preparations. J. Clin. Invest. *38*:1022, 1959.

582. HEATHCOTE, J. G., AND MOONEY, F. S.: The oral treatment of pernicious anemia. Lancet *1*:982, 1958.

583. NYBERG, W., AND REIZENSTEIN, P.: Intestinal absorption of radiovitamin B_{12} bound in pig liver. Lancet *2*:832, 1958.

584. CASTLE, W. B.: Oral treatment of pernicious anemia. Lancet *2*:270, 1958.

585. LATNER, A. L.: Absorption of bound radioactive vitamin B_{12}. Lancet *2*:961, 1958.

586. GRÄSBECK, R., RUNEBERG, L., SIMONS, K., AND NYBERG, W.: Absorption of bound radioactive vitamin B_{12}. Lancet *2*:961, 1958.

587. CHOW, B. F., MEIER, P., AND FREE, S. M.: Absorption of vitamin B_{12} enhanced by d-sorbitol. Am. J. Clin. Nutrition. *6*:30, 1958.

588. HERBERT, V., BIERFASS, M., WASSERMAN, L. R., ESTREN, S., AND BRODY, E.: Effect of d-sorbitol on absorption of vitamin B_{12} by human subjects able to produce intrinsic factor. Am. J. Clin. Nutrition. *7*:325, 1959.

589. ELLENBOGEN, L., HERBERT, V., AND WILLIAMS, W. L.: Effect of d-sorbitol on absorption of vitamin B_{12} by pernicious anemia patients. Proc. Soc. Exper. Biol. & Med. *99*:257, 1958.

590. CHALMERS, J. N. M., AND SHINTON, N. K.: Effect of d-sorbitol on the absorption of orally administered vitamin B_{12}. Nature *183*:118, 1959.

591. HERBERT, V.: Sorbitol and vitamin B_{12} absorption. Am. J. Clin. Nutrition. *6*:547, 1958.

592. The Pharmacopeia of the United States of America, Fifteenth Revision. Official from December 15, 1955.

593. JUKES, T. H.: B-Vitamins for Blood Formation. Springfield, Ill., Charles C Thomas, 1952.

594. SCHOENBACH, E. B., GREENSPAN, E. M., AND COLSKY, J.: Reversal of Aminopterin and Amethopterin toxicity by citrovorum factor. J.A.M.A. *144*:1558, 1950.

595. CONDIT, P. T., AND GROB, D.: Studies on the folic acid vitamins. I. Observa-

tions on the metabolism of folic acid in man and on the effect of aminopterin. Cancer *11*:525, 1958.

596. JUKES, T. H.: Recent studies with hemopoietic factors, intrinsic factor, and folic acid. *In* Proceedings of the Sixth International Congress of the International Society of Hematology. New York, Grune & Stratton, 1958.

597. NOREN, B.: Allergic reactions in parenteral liver therapy, and vitamin B_{12}. Acta med. scandinav. *137*:48, 1950.

598. OSTLING, G., NYBERG, W., AND GORDIN, R.: Antianemic activity of alkali-treated crude liver extract. Acta med. scandinav. *145*:40, 1953.

599. OWREN, P. A.: A protein synthesis liver factor lacking in pernicious anemia and related macrocytic anemias. Scandinav. J. Clin. & Lab. Invest. *2*:241, 1950.

600. ———: Is B_{12} the complete therapeutic answer in pernicious anemia? *In* Proceedings of the Third International Congress of the International Society of Hematology. New York, Grune & Stratton, 1951.

601. GORDIN, R.: Prothrombin in cryptogenic pernicious anemia and pernicious tapeworm anemia and its response to treatment. Acta med. scandinav. *149*:1, 1954.

602. BEZMAN, A., KINNEAR, D. G., AND ZAMCHECK, N.: D-xylose and potassium iodide absorption and serum carotene in pernicious anemia. J. Lab. & Clin. Med. *53*:226, 1959.

603. SPAET, T. H., AND KROPATKIN, M.: Studies on "prothrombin derivatives" in vitamin K deficiency. A. M. A. Arch. Int. Med. *102*:558, 1958.

604. WANG, C. I., AND BOSSAK, E. T.: Hemorrhagic manifestations in idiopathic sprue: a report of 25 cases and review of the literature. J. Mount Sinai Hosp. (New York) *24*:317, 1957. Simultaneously published in Adlersberg, D.: The Malabsorption Syndrome. New York, Grune & Stratton, 1957.

605. VILTER, R. W.: Ascorbic acid deficiency (scurvy). *In* Harrison, T. R., Adams, R. D., Bennett, I. L., Jr., Resnik, W. H., Thorn, G. W., and Wintrobe, M. M.: Principles of Internal Medicine. New York, McGraw-Hill, 1958.

606. ———: Ascorbic acid. IX. Effects of deficiency in human beings. *In* Sebrell, W. H. Jr., and Harris, R. S.: The Vitamins. New York. Academic Press, 1954, vol. 1.

607. ———: Ascorbic acid. XI (B). Requirements of human beings. *In* Sebrell, W. H., Jr., and Harris, R. S.: The Vitamins. New York, Academic Press, 1954, vol. 1.

608. COX, E. V., GADDIE, R., MATTHEWS, D., COOKE, W. T., AND MEYNELL, M. J.: An inter-relationship between ascorbic acid and cyanocobalamin. Clin. Sc. *17*:681, 1958.

609. WALLERSTEIN, R. O., HARRIS, J. W., AND GABUZDA, G. J.: Ascorbic acid deficiency in pernicious anemia. Am. J. Med. *14*:532, 1953.

610. CROSBY, W. H.: Misuse of blood transfusion. Blood *13*:1198, 1958.

611. ADLERSBERG, D., COLCHER, H., AND WANG, C.: Oral use of hydrocortisone (Compound F) in treatment of sprue. Arch. Int. Med. *92*:615, 1953.

612. WOLLAEGER, E. E.: Sprue and allied malabsorption syndromes. *In* CECIL, R. L., AND LOEB, R. F., EDS.: A Textbook of Medicine, ed. 10, Philadelphia, W. B. Saunders, 1959.

Index

Achlorhydria. *See also* Gastric acidity
  combined iron and B12 deficiency with, 14
  determination by tubeless methods, 80–81
    erroneous results in, 80–81
  pernicious anemia without, 23, 80
  pernicious anemia and, 22–25, 79–81
Acid and vitamin B12 absorption, 30
Addison, Sir Thomas, 21, 63
  pernicious anemia described by, 63
Addison's disease in association with pernicious anemia, 26
Addisonian pernicious anemia, 22–25. *See also* Pernicious anemia.
Adrenocortical steroids. *See* Steroids.
Adrenocorticotrophic hormone treatment in malabsorption syndrome, 108, 114–115
  in coeliac disease, 114
  in tropical sprue, 32, 114
Aging
  increased incidence of gastric atrophy with, 2
  megaloblastic anemia with, 2, 20
  poor diet with, 20
  serum vitamin B12 lower with, 2
Agranulocytosis, 60, 61
Alcoholism, chronic
  folic acid deficiency with, 19, 52–53, 76
  vitamin B12 deficiency with, 19
Aminopterin-produced megaloblastic anemia, 56
  treatment, 56, 110
Amytal, producing megaloblastic anemia, 56
Anastomosis, intestine, producing megaloblastic anemia, 34, 40. *See also* Blind loop syndrome.
Anemia
  achrestic, 59–60
Addisonian pernicious. *See* Pernicious anemia.
  aplastic, 61–62
    macrocytes in, 12, 61
    resulting from untreated megaloblastic anemia, 61–62, 98–99
  aregenerative, 61
  blood transfusion in, 113–114
  dimorphic, 12
  fish tapeworm pernicious. *See* Fish tapeworm megaloblastic anemia.
  hemolytic
    megaloblastic anemia in, 60, 61, 74, 78
    pernicious anemia as, 75
    reticulocytosis from folic acid in, in presence of normoblastic bone marrow, 61. *See also* Hemoglobin synthesis, defective, masking megaloblastic anemia.
  idiopathic refractory megaloblastic. *See* Achrestic anemia.

  macrocytic. *See also* Megaloblastic anemia.
    in aplastic anemia, 12
    in liver disease, 12, 52–53
      cirrhosis, 52–53
    refractory, 59
    tropical and nontropical, 51–52
  megaloblastic. *See* Megaloblastic anemia.
  nutritional megaloblastic. *See* Nutritional megaloblastic anemia.
  pernicious. *See* Pernicious anemia.
  refractory
    macrocytic, 59
    megaloblastic, 59–62
      folic acid deficiency in, 59–60
      orotic aciduria in, 62
      steroid treatment of, 62
      vitamin B6 deficiency in, 61
      yeast extract treatment of, 62
    normoblastic, 60
Anisocytosis, 3
  producing macrocytes, 12
Antagonists. *See* Antimetabolites.
Anthelminthics for fish tapeworm infestation, 104, 115
Antibiotic treatment
  in blind loop syndrome, 40, 115
  in megaloblastic anemia, 40
  in pernicious anemia, 40, 115
  in tropical sprue, 54
Anticonvulsant-produced megaloblastic anemia, 56–58
  folic acid for, 56
  vitamin B12 for, 56
  withdrawal of anticonvulsant for, 56
Antimetabolites
  of folic acid, 56–57, 110–111
  of pyrimidines, 57
  of thymine, 57
  of vitamin B12, 41
Anti-pernicious anemia principle, 21, 22
Anti-vitamin B12, 41
  in treatment of malignancies, 41
Arneth count shift to the right, 6, 9. *See also* Neutrophils, hypersegmented.
  early sign of megaloblastic anemia, 7–10, 52–53, 66–68, 69–70, 77, 85, 105, 110
Artery, superior mesenteric, occlusion of, 34, 35
  producing defective vitamin B12 absorption, 35
  resection producing defective vitamin B12 absorption, 34
Ascaris lumbricoides, 39
Ascorbic acid
  content of milk, 46